TEACHINGS OF
TIBETAN
YOGA

TEACHINGS OF TIBETAN YOGA

translated and annotated by
GARMA C. C. CHANG

A Citadel Press Book
Published by Carol Publishing Group

Published by agreement with INSTITUTE FOR INNER STUDIES, INC.

A Citadel Press Book
Published by Carol Publishing Group
Citadel Press is a registered trademark of Carol Communications, Inc.

Editorial Offices: 600 Madison Avenue, New York, NY 10022
Sales & Distribution Offices: 120 Enterprise Avenue, Secaucus, NJ 07094
In Canada: Canadian Manda Group, P.O. Box 920, Station U, Toronto,
Ontario, M8Z 5P9, Canada

Queries regarding rights and permissions should be addressed to:
Carol Publishing Group, 600 Madison Avenue, New York, NY 10022

Manufactured in the United States of America
ISBN 0-8065-1453-1

Carol Publishing Group books are available at special discounts
for bulk purchases, for sales promotions, fund raising, or
educational purposes. Special editions can also be created to
specifications. For details contact: Special Sales Department,
Carol Publishing Group, 120 Enterprise Ave., Secaucus, NJ 07094

By the same author:

THE PRACTICE OF ZEN
Harper & Row, 1959

THE HUNDRED THOUSAND SONGS OF MILAREPA
University Books, 1962

Introduction

The author-translator of this book was born in China into a highly-placed family some forty years ago. In early youth he broke out of this pattern to become the disciple of a Buddhist Guru, in a part of China near Tibet. His Guru sent him to Tibet to further his training. After eight years in Tibetan monasteries, six of them under one Guru, he came West to study animal husbandry and to bring this knowledge back to Tibet. The Communist victory in China and the Communist invasion of Tibet cut him off from return. His devotion to Tibetan Buddhism can now best be expressed by translating into English the unknown teachings of Tibetan Buddhism. Last year he gave us the first complete translation of *The Hundred Thousand Songs of Milarepa,* the principal religious work of Tibet. Now he gives us, in a short and extremely concentrated book, an introduction to the spiritual, mental, and physical exercises of his religion. He is writing not only as a Chinese Buddhist scholar telling us about the Tibetan variety of Buddhism but, even more, as a Chinese who has become a Tibetan Buddhist. He has sought to make this fact precise by giving up his original Chinese name, Chen-chi Chang, and adopting a Tibetan name, Garma C. C. Chang. This book is most profitably read, then, not as a scholarly work but as an introduction to a religion by which its author-translator lives.

Furthermore, this book will most profitably be read by those Westerners who have really left behind denominational parochialism. To put it quite plainly, we are publishing this book for an audience of educated laymen in the Western world who have ceased to be Christian, at least in any traditional sense. We are publishing this book for the

reader who understands that all the great religions belong
to him as part of his human past, that he "belongs" to
none of them. In the very helpful words of the Reverend
Kenneth L. Patton, of Boston's Charles Street Universalist
Meeting House:

"The role of appreciation in the religious experience is
strangely neglected amongst us. We seem to believe that our
religion consists only of those precepts and attitudes that
we practice. And yet, we can appreciate a great wealth of
human experience and attitudes which we never would care
to practice ourselves. I would try to appreciate *everything* in
man's religious history. In this sense, I would seek to be a
complete universalist. And I believe that my critical and
intuitive selection from the human and natural scene of
those elements that will become my *practicing* religion will
depend on whether my appreciation has attained universal
scope. Otherwise, it would proceed from ignorance and
prejudice and would be worth little."

If the reader will firmly keep in mind that he is first seek-
ing to *appreciate* as fully and completely as possible the
religion of Tibetan Buddhism, quite independently of
whether he will ever care to practice any of it, he will get
the most out of his first reading of this book. Open yourself
to it and let it take possession of you!

Part I of this book is relatively easy to understand and
relatively familiar. It is sufficiently similar to some kinds of
Western religion.

Part II is much more important and much more difficult
to understand. It is to center attention on it that we have
titled this book *Teachings of Tibetan Yoga*, that is, to
emphasize the *practice* of the Yoga exercises.

Most readers, even those who have read a good deal
about Yoga, will find the practice of Dumo—the generating

of internal heat in one's body – strange and not at all easy to believe. I want to call to the reader's attention the fact that this Dumo is the very foundation of the whole of Tibetan Yoga, without which no other part of it makes the slightest sense. That makes it all the harder to believe. Nevertheless, there it is. As it is presented here, its practice and its meaning are quite peculiar to Tantric Buddhism. But for varying meanings, the generating of internal heat as part of religious practice goes back for tens of thousands of years. The reader who wishes to pursue this extraordinary subject further will find it dealt with in Mircea Eliade's monumental work, *Shamanism.*

Dumo's special meaning for Tibetan Yoga flows from the profoundly anti-ascetic and anti-pessimistic doctrine of Tantric Buddhism. The author-translator has made a great effort, in his Foreword, to provide a bridge for Western readers to understand Tibetan Tantrism. Please read his Foreword most carefully. He means precisely what he says when he tells you that opposites are also inseparable unities and that the best example of this is that the human body-mind can be made into the body of Buddha. I suppose that for Westerners the most difficult example of all is that sexual bliss can become divine bliss. The author-translator is justly fearful of being misunderstood on this crucial question of erotic mysticism. As to the actual practices, he has provided the texts intact but it may well be that his notes leave certain questions unanswered which must be most puzzling to Westerners.

As in the case of Dumo, the retention in the body of male semen has a special meaning in Tantrism, although this idea (and practice) has an age-long history. In ancient Hindu and Chinese medicine, among other archaic medi-cines, it is believed that orgasm without ejaculation is not only heathful but preserves the semen and leads to long life. Modern physiology has not yet found any evidence of this kind, for orgasm without ejaculation in a normal person results simply in the semen being discharged into the bladder. Today we cannot know whether the original author of the Six Yogas understood the actual physiology, but we can be quite certain that Mr. Chang does. The point is that the Tig Le retention continues to be crucial to Tibetan Tantrism because here the practice is based not on a mistaken physiology but on a mystical technique: in effect, *all* the life processes are reversed, turned topsy-turvy, taken out of the realm of nature: breathing is stopped as far as possible, thinking stopped, hearing stopped, seeing stopped, and so on — in a word, everything is transformed. I do not pretend that this is a doctrine easy to understand, and it should be obvious that even more difficult is it a practice to achieve — and Mr. Chang warns you sternly not to try it without the help of a Guru. But, at least, please understand that it is not a matter of outmoded physiology.

All I am trying to do in this Introduction is to make it a little easier for Western readers to understand Mr. Chang's book. When he speaks of "Tantric physiology," he does not mean a physiology subject to scientific verification. There have been many attempts to identify the Cakra centers with the actual human physiology, and, again, it may be that the ancient yogis thought of it as actual physiology. But Mr. Chang knows better.

I am afraid that Mr. Chang's notes do not provide Westerners with much light on the numerous references to male-female relationships in the Six Yogas. The Dakinis, the female deities of Tantrism, Mr. Chang tells us "protect and serve the Tantric Doctrine. They are not invariably enlightened beings; there are many so-called Worldly

Dakinis," but here he ends. What is involved, I think, is Mr. Chang's anxiety not to cheapen or sensationalize Tantrism. It may be, too, that he assumes we will understand the implications of the anti-ascetic doctrine that male-female, "though apparently antithetical, is, in reality, an inseparable unity." Nevertheless, a number of passages in the Six Yogas cannot but be puzzling to a good many Western readers, for example, such a passage as: "If these measures still fail to produce a Great Bliss, one may apply the *Wisdom-Mother Mudra* by visualizing the sexual act with a Dakini . . ." The reader should understand that what is involved is of course sexual intercourse but in a context like that described above dealing with Tig Le: the woman must truly be consecrated as a goddess, she must really become a goddess, just as the disciple becomes a Buddha. It is not a figure of speech any more than the yogi's successful reduction of the rate of his heartbeat, or his ceasing to hear, see, or know anything other than the Great Bliss. Beyond these few words of explanation, nothing more is really necessary for reading Mr. Chang's book. The truly interested reader will be well rewarded, even though, inevitably, more than one passage in it will remain an utter mystery to him. There was a time when the learned well knew that no really worthwhile book would be fully understood even at a third reading. Why should this not be so?

* * *

The congregational religions of the Western world provide very little preparation through which to understand the religion that Mr. Chang practices. Most of the "practice" of a congregational religion consists in sitting quite passively as part of a considerable number of persons, while a priest or minister officiates. Whatever is not passive is usually done together, as singing hymns, or praying aloud. The principal exception to this situation is to say one's prayers alone, as at night. How little of this goes on, and how perfunctorily, after childhood, is quite well known, I think. There is, however, another kind of exception, and that is the class of individuals whom we term mystics, who break out of the congregational passivity, and practice religion on their own, and, indeed, of their own. It is notable, and significant, that most mystics are considered "mavericks," and at best are in a state of uneasy truce with the officials of any Western church.

In one of his attempts to find a bridge to Western readers, Mr. Chang seeks to define Tibetan Tantrism as a mysticism. This may help some Westerners understand it better, thanks to the active role of mystics, but the Tibetan mystic does not have to pay the price of uneasy truce with the officials of his religion. On the contrary, his closest relationship, usually lasting a lifetime, is with his Guru.

The point is that we are in the presence of a kind of religion where analogies are few and not very helpful. Mr. Chang explains in his Foreword that it is not his aim to make a critical study of Tibetan Tantrism versus other forms of mysticism. It was a wise decision, for it could not have been fruitful. In a word, dear reader, grasp the nettle; you must get at Tibetan Tantrism for what it is, because what it is is worth knowing, precisely because it is so unique.

JOHN C. WILSON

New York, N. Y.
December, 1962

Foreword

If mysticism is defined, in its broader sense, as "the Doctrine that direct knowledge of 'God' or spiritual truth is attainable through immediate intuition," Tibetan Tantrism can also be considered as a form of mysticism. The problem here is, of course, in what sense to understand the terms "knowledge," "God," "spiritual truth," and "intuition." A careful analysis of the use of these words will immediately bring into the open the complex and divergent concepts behind them, and no generally agreed understanding seems to be at hand. Despite the apparent similarity of the various forms of mysticism, great differences do exist between them. But to point out the differences in detail, a thorough knowledge of all these systems is needed, together with personal experience of each of them as verified by scores of mystics. These requirements are indeed too difficult, if not impossible, for any individual to fulfill today. The author's aim is not, therefore, to make a critical study of Tibetan Tantrism *versus* other forms of mysticism, but to introduce to the general reader several important texts hitherto unavailable in European languages.

A few words about the basic doctrine of Tibetan Tantrism and the fundamental principle that underlies its practice may be helpful. It can be summarized in the following words: "The divinity of Buddhahood is omnipresent, but the quickest way to realize this truth is to discover it within one's body-mind complex." By spiritual exercises and the application of Tantric techniques—such as the Six Yogas—one can soon realize that his body, mind, and the "objective world" are all manifestations of the divine Buddha-hood. Samsara is Nirvana, men are "gods," the "impure" passion-desires are themselves expressions of the Five Innate Buddhas,[1] Enlightenment or Liberation is not attained by eradicating man's passion-desires but by identifying them with the transcendental Wisdom. The basic doctrine of Tibetan Tantrism can thus be called a doctrine of viewing man's body-mind complex as corresponding to, if not identical with, that of Buddha. The spirit and practice of all Tantric Yogas are also directed toward the unfoldment of this basic principle.

Now, let us take the two pillars of Tantric practice, the Arising and Perfecting Yogas, as illustrations for this basic doctrine. In the Arising Yoga practice, the yogi is taught to visualize and thus identify the outer world as Mandalas; his body as the Body of the Patron Buddha; his nervous system as the Three Channels and the nadis of the four Cakras; his secretions as the bindus of the positive and negative elements; his aspiration and energy as the Wisdom-Prana and "Light". . . . In the Perfecting Yoga practice he is taught first to dissolve all his Energy-Thought[2] in the Innate Light—the Dharmakaya—hitherto concealed "in" the Center of the Heart Cakra, and from it again to project the Body-of-Form (Rupakaya), and thus to animate the infinite acts of Buddhahood.

An important theory, underlying the practice of Tibetan Yogas, called "The Identity of Prana and Mind"[3] should also be mentioned here. Tantrism views the world as consisting of contrasting, antithetical elements and relationships: noumenon and phenomenon, potentiality and manifestation, reason and affect, Nirvana and Samsara . . . *Prana and Mind*. Each of these dualities, though apparently antithetical, is, in reality, an inseparable unity. If one can understand completely and master one member of the duality, he automatically understands and masters the other. Thus, he who realizes the essence of mind as being Transcendental Wisdom will at the same time realize the essence of prana as being inexhaustible vitality and the act of Buddhahood. It is not necessary to expound here all the many aspects of this doctrine, but one of the more important of them should receive some attention, namely "the reciprocal character of mind and prana." This means that a certain type of mind, or mental activity, is invariably accompanied by a prana of corresponding character, whether transcendental or mundane. For instance, a particular mood, feeling, or thought is always accompanied by a prana of corresponding character and rhythm which is reflected in the phenomenon of breathing. Thus anger produces not merely an inflamed thought-feeling, but also a harsh and accentuated "roughness" of breathing. On the other hand, when there is calm concentration on an intellectual problem, the thought and the breathing exhibit a like calmness. When the concentration is deep, as during an effort to solve a subtle problem, unconsciously the breath is held. When one is in a mood of anger, pride, envy, shame, arrogance, love, lust, and so on, this particular "prana" or "air" can be felt immediately within oneself. In deep Samadhi no thought arises, so there is no perceptible breathing. At the initial moment of Enlightenment, when normal consciousness is transformed, the prana undergoes a revolutionary change. Accordingly, every mood, thought, and feeling—whether simple, subtle, or complex—is accompanied by a corresponding or reciprocal prana. In the advanced stage of Dhyana, the circulation of the blood is slowed down almost to cessation, perceptible breathing also ceases, and the yogi experiences some degree of illumination in a thought-free state of mind. Then not only will a change of consciousness occur, but also a change in the physiological functioning of the body.

Basing itself upon this principle, Tibetan Tantrism offers two Paths, or types of Yoga, both leading to the same supramundane goal. One is called the Path of Liberation, or "Mind Yoga," and the other, the Path of Skillfulness or "Energy Yoga." The former is in many ways like Ch'an (Zen) Buddhism because it stresses the observation and cultivation of the Innate Mind, and requires only a minimum of ritual and yogic preparations. The latter is a series of rigorous and complex Yoga practices known as the Arising and Perfecting Yogas. The three excerpts dealing with Mahamudra in the first part of this book are of the former group, which the reader may soon discover to be strikingly similiar to early Zen Buddhism. The Six Yogas of Naropa are of the latter group—a synthesis of the Arising and Perfecting Yogas, with special emphasis on the latter.

From the yogic viewpoint, among the group of the Six Yogas those of the Heat and Illusory Body are the primary ones, and the other four: Dream, Light, Bardo, and Transformation, are ramifications of them. Nevertheless, for those who are interested in studying the "unconscious" and "superconscious" states, the Dream and Light Yogas may be more important, because they give essential information on the subject. To provide readers with a general background to the Six Yogas, an epitome of Lama Drashi Namjhal's Introduction to them—a simple but clear text—is translated. Because at this time the translator has no access to the original Tibetan texts, the three Mahamudra excerpts and

Drashi Namjhal's *Six Yogas* are translated from Chinese versions recently secured from Buddhist sources in Hongkong and Taiwan.[4] All diacritical marks in romanized Tibetan and Sanskrit words have been omitted in the text, since they would only confuse and distract general readers and are unnecessary for the specialist who will at once recognize the original Tibetan and Sanskrit words. But in the Notes and Glossary, these diacritical marks are incorporated for easier identification of the more important terms. Definitions and explanations of a few dozen of the most commonly used terms appearing in the text, are given in the Glossary to assist new readers.

The translator declines all responsibility for readers who may rashly experiment with these Six Yogas. A mere reading of these texts can never replace a living Guru from whom a serious Bodhi-seeker should first receive initiation and guidance before he can start the actual practice. For serious students, this book can serve no more than as a source of reference, a pointer to the Way.

The translator, fearful lest these important teachings be lost in their mother-land under the tyranny of Communism, has broken with tradition by revealing these hitherto "secretly guarded" documents in English translation, with the hope that they may prove useful to seekers of truth.

GARMA C. C. CHANG

Madison, Wisconsin
December, 1962

NOTES

1 The Five Innate Buddhas: Vairocana, Aksobhya, Ratnasaṁbhava, Amitābha, Amoghasiddhi. They represent the sublimation of ignorance, of hatred, of pride, of lust and of envy. They are also mistakenly called the "Five Dhyāna Buddhas"—as they appear in the five directions in a Maṇḍala symbolizing the innate Buddha nature within oneself.

2 Energy-Thought, or Prāṇa-Mind (T.T.: Rluñ.Sems.): According to Tantrism, prāṇa—that which acts: the energy, and mind— that which knows: the consciousness, are two aspects of one entity, inseparable and interdependent. See the explanations of the "Identity of Mind and Prāṇa" theory in the next paragraph of the Foreword.

3 The explanations here given are quoted, with some minor alterations, from the translator's "Yogic Commentary," in Evans-Wentz' *Tibetan Yoga and Secret Doctrines,* 2nd edition, Oxford University Press, 1958.

4 The Chinese translation of Drashi Namjhal's *Six Yogas* was made by Mang Kung; of *The Song of Mahāmudrā,* by Fa Tsun; *The Vow of Mahāmudrā,* by Garma C. C. Chang; and *The Essentials of Mahāmudrā,* by Mr. Chang's Guru, the Venerable Lama Kong Ka.

Glossary

1 Ālaya Consciousness—the Store Consciousness which preserves the "seeds" of mental impressions and supports the formation of habit. Memory and learning are made possible because of this Consciousness. It is the Foundation or "root" of the other Consciousnesses, and is regarded by some Schools of Mahāyāna Buddhism as the "Primordial," or "Universal" Consciousness.

2 Arising and Perfecting Yogas—the two main Yoga practices of Tibetan Tantrism. Arising Yoga is the "Yoga of Growth or Creation"; Perfecting Yoga is the "Yoga of Consummation." See the Foreword.

3 Bardo—the intermediate stage between death and rebirth.

4 Bīja, meaning "seed" (T.T.: Sa.Bon.)—a special sound or syllable which is believed to represent the essence of a deity, a principle, a Cakra, or the like.

5 Bindu (lit.: "drop" or "dot"; T.T.: Thig.Le.)—In Tibetan Tantrism, Bindu or Tig Le usually refers to the essence of the vital energy of the body, especially male semen. Tig Le in "Tantric physiology" seems to refer to the secretions of the endocrine system.

6 Bodhi—that of Buddha, or that which concerns Buddhahood.

7 Bodhi-Mind (Skt.: Bodhicitta)—the aspiration to Buddhahood, the "thought of Enlightenment," the insight into immanent reality, the great compassion and Vow to serve, benefit, and deliver all sentient beings. In Tantrism, this term is used to denote the Tig Le—semen and endocrine secretions—thus implying its hidden connection with Compassion and Wisdom.

8 Bodhisattva—a man who has taken a vow to strive for Enlightenment and save all sentient beings; a man who aspires to Buddha-

17

hood and altruistic deeds; an enlightened being, or a follower of Mahāyāna Buddhism.

9 Cakra—a psychic center, or a Center of the nādīs in Tantric physiology.

10 Central Channel (T.T.: rTsa.dBu.Ma.)—the main Channel that leads to Nirvāṇa, situated in the center of the "Yogic Body." All Saṃsāric energies and thoughts are to be converted to transcendental Wisdom and Power within this Channel.

11 Ḍākinīs—goddesses, or female deities of Tantrism.

12 Devas—gods, angels, heavenly beings.

13 Dharma—This term has three major usages in Buddhism:
   (1) Buddhist Doctrine, or teachings;
   (2) object, being, or matter; and
   (3) principles or laws.

14 Dharmakāya—the "Body of Truth," or the "Real" Body of Buddha, which is formless, omnipresent, ultimate, void, and yet all-embracing.

15 Dhyāna—an equivalent of Samādhi which, according to the Buddhist doctrine, denotes a group of pure concentrative states.

16 Dumo (T.T.: gTum.Mo.)—the "mystic fire" produced in the Navel Center through the practice of Heat Yoga.

17 Experience and Realization (T.T.: Ñams. [and] rTog.Pa.)—Experience denotes the incomplete and imperfect, yet genuine mystic experience a yogi attains in meditation; Realization is the complete, clear, and perfect mystic experience.

18 Mahāmudrā (lit., the Great Symbol)—a teaching that leads to the realization of the Primordial Mind, or the Dharmakāya; the practical instructions on how to meditate on Śūnyatā (Voidness).

19 Maṇḍala (T.T.: dKyil.hKhor.)—meaning "circle" or "center."
The Maṇḍala is a symbolic, geometrical diagram representing
the phenomenal world of Tantric Buddhas. It is a "center" or
realm wherein the Tantric deities dwell.

20 Māyā—the Doctrine that all phenomena and experiences in the
manifested universe are illusions or magic plays; that all matter
is devoid of self-entity.

21 Nāḍīs—the "psychic nerves" that transmit the vital energies; the
mystical "channels" within the Yogic Body.

22 Nirmāṇakāya—the Transformation Body of Buddha, which in-
carnates in numerous forms in the various worlds.

23 Nirvāṇa—the state of ultimate Liberation.

24 Pāramitās—the spiritual deeds of a Bodhisattva; the meritorious
and altruistic actions that enable one to reach the state of Perfect
Enlightenment.

25 Prāṇa—This term conveys many meanings, such as air, breath,
energy, vital force, and so forth. In this text it usually denotes
either (1) the breath, or (2) the "air-" or energy-currents of
the body.

26 Prāṇa-Mind (T.T.: Rluṅ.Sems.)—According to Tibetan Tantrism,
mind and prāṇa are two facets of one entity—they should never
be treated as two separate things. Mind is that which is aware;
prāṇa is the active energy which gives support to this awareness.
He who masters the mind, automatically masters the prāṇa, and
vice versa.

27 Samādhi—literally meaning "putting together" or "combining
with," i.e., a pure or "transic" concentrative state wherein the
mind and the observed object are merged into one.

28 Sambhogakāya—the glorious and divine body of Buddha, manifested in the Pure Land and visible only to enlightened Bodhisattvas.

29 Samsāra—the doctrine of reincarnation; the continual round of birth-and-death.

30 Śūnyatā—Voidness or Emptiness; the doctrine that all becomings in the phenomenal world are devoid of self-nature, entity, or substance—that they are illusorily existent but not truly so; that which denies all the views based on existence or non-existence, being or non-being.

31 Tantras—the holy Scriptures of Tantrism.

32 Trikāya—the Three Bodies of Buddhahood, i.e., the Dharmakāya, the Body of Truth; the Sambhogakāya, the Divine Body, or the Body of Enjoyment; Nirmāṇakāya, the Transformation or Incarnated Body.

33 Tig Le (T.T.: Thig.Le.; Skt.: Bindu)—the vital source of physical energy, i.e., semen, secretions of the endocrine system, and the like.

Contents

Part I

The Teaching
of Mahamudra

The Song
of Mahamudra[1]

by
Tilopa

Mahamudra is beyond all words
And symbols, but for you, Naropa,
Earnest and loyal, must this be said.

The Void needs no reliance,
Mahamudra rests on nought.
Without making an effort,
But remaining loose and natural,
One can break the yoke
Thus gaining Liberation.

If one sees nought when staring into space,
If with the mind one then observes the mind,
One destroys distinctions
And reaches Buddhahood.

The clouds that wander through the sky
Have no roots, no home; nor do the distinctive
Thoughts floating through the mind.
Once the Self-mind is seen,
Discrimination stops.

In space shapes and colors form,
But neither by black nor white is space tinged.
From the Self-mind all things emerge, the mind
By virtues and by vices is not stained.

The darkness of ages cannot shroud
The glowing sun; the long kalpas
Of Samsara ne'er can hide
The Mind's brilliant light.

Though words are spoken to explain the Void,
The Void as such can never be expressed.
Though we say "the mind is a bright light,"
It is beyond all words and symbols.
Although the mind is void in essence,
All things it embraces and contains.

Do nought with the body but relax,
Shut firm the mouth and silent remain,
Empty your mind and think of nought.
Like a hollow bamboo
Rest at ease your body.
Giving not nor taking,
Put your mind at rest.
Mahamudra is like a mind that clings to nought.
Thus practicing, in time you will reach Buddhahood.

The practice of Mantra and Paramita,
Instruction in the Sutras and Precepts,
And teaching from the Schools and Scriptures
    will not bring
Realization of the Innate Truth.

For if the mind when filled with some desire
Should seek a goal, it only hides the Light.

He who keeps Tantric Precepts
Yet discriminates, betrays
The spirit of Samaya.[2]
Cease all activity, abandon
All desire, let thoughts rise and fall
As they will like the ocean waves.
He who never harms the Non-abiding
Nor the Principle of Non-distinction,
Upholds the Tantric Precepts.

He who abandons craving
And clings not to this or that,
Perceives the real meaning
Given in the Scriptures.

In Mahamudra all one's sins are burned;
In Mahamudra one is released
From the prison of this world.
This is the Dharma's supreme torch.
Those who disbelieve it
Are fools who ever wallow
In misery and sorrow.

To strive for Liberation
One should rely on a Guru.
When your mind receives his blessing
Emancipation is at hand.

Alas, all things in this world are meaningless,
They are but sorrow's seeds.
Small teachings lead to acts;
One should only follow
Teachings that are great.

To transcend duality
Is the Kingly View;
To conquer distractions is
The Royal Practice;
The Path of No-practice
Is the Way of Buddhas;
He who treads that Path
Reaches Buddhahood.

Transient is this world;
Like phantoms and dreams,
Substance it has none.
Renounce it and forsake your kin,
Cut the strings of lust and hatred,
Meditate in woods and mountains.
If without effort you remain
Loosely in the "natural state,"
Soon Mahamudra you will win
And attain the Non-attainment.

Cut the root of a tree
And the leaves will wither;
Cut the root of your mind
And Samsara falls.

The light of any lamp
Dispels in a moment
The darkness of long kalpas;
The strong light of the mind
In but a flash will burn
The veil of ignorance.

Whoever clings to mind sees not
The truth of what's Beyond the mind.
Whoever *strives* to practice Dharma
Finds *not* the truth of Beyond-practice.
To know what is Beyond both mind and practice,
One should cut cleanly through the root of mind
And stare naked. One should thus break away
From all distinctions and remain at ease.

One should not give or take
But remain natural,
For Mahamudra is beyond
All acceptance and rejection.
Since the Alaya³ is not born,
No one can obstruct or soil it;
Staying in the "Unborn" realm
All appearance will dissolve
Into the Dharmata,⁴ all self-will
And pride will vanish into nought.

The supreme Understanding transcends
All this and that. The supreme Action
Embraces great resourcefulness
Without attachment. The supreme
Accomplishment is to realize
Immanence without hope.

At first a yogi feels his mind
Is tumbling like a waterfall;
In mid-course, like the Ganges
It flows on slow and gentle;
In the end, it is a great
Vast ocean, where the Lights
Of Son and Mother[5] merge in one.

The Vow
of Mahamudra[1]

by

Garmapa Rangjang Dorje

(1)

In the Mandala I see the Guru, Yidam, and Holy Beings,
In all times and directions I see the Buddhas
   and Bodhisattvas,
With deep sincerity to you all I pray;
Pray bless my good wishes with Accomplishment!

(2)

The good deeds of mind and body
And the virtues of all beings
Are pure and clear streams from the Snow Mountain.
In freedom may they flow down to the sea
Of the Four Bodies of Buddhahood.[2]

(3)

Through all my lives in future times
May I not hear words like
"Pain" and "sin." May I always
Share joy and goodness
In the vast Dharma sea.

(4)

May I always have leisure, faith, diligence, and wisdom,
Meet good Gurus and receive their Pith-Instructions.
In my practice may I never meet
With hindrances, but e'er enjoy
The Dharma in my future lives.

31

(5)

May the Rational and Holy Judgements[3]
Liberate me from ignorance; may
The Pith-Instructions destroy all doubt
And darkness. Through the light of meditation
May I vividly behold the naked Truth,
And kindle the Light of the Three Wisdoms!

(6)

The Principle is the Two-Truths[4] beyond
The views of positive and negative;
The Path is the spiritual preparation
Outstripping both increase and decrease;
The Accomplishment is the Two-Benefits[5]
Transcending both Samsara and Nirvana.
May I always meet with these right
Teachings throughout my future lives!

(7)

Mind-Essence is void and radiant—
The real source of Two-in-One.
The diamond-cutter Mahamudra
Purifies. The purified
Are ignorance and vices—
Momentary confusions.
May I attain the immaculate Dharmakaya—
The fruit of being purified.

(8)

The View of Mahamudra is to add
Nothing to Mind's nature. Being mindful
Of this View, without distraction, is the
Essence of Practice. Of all practices,
This is the supreme one. May I attain
The Teaching of the View and Practice.

(9)

All forms are but expressions of one's mind;
The mind is of no-mind and void in nature.
Though void, 'tis not extinct,
But manifests all things.
May I always observe this Truth
And attain a decisive View.

(10)

Confused, self-manifestations that are void
We deem to be real objects and outside ourselves;
We hold self-awareness
To be our true Ego.
Because of these Two Clingings,[6]
Men wander in Samsara.
O, may I cut off
The root blindness!

(11)

"Nothing really is!" For even
Buddha no existence sees.
"All is not empty!" For Nirvana
And Samsara do exist.
This wondrous Middle Way of Two-in-One is neither
In harmony nor conflict. O, may I realize
The Self-mind which is free from all discriminations.

(12)

No one can describe *That* by saying "It is this!"
No one can deny *That* by saying "It's not this!"
This non-being of the real Dharma
Which transcends the realm of Consciousness—
May I understand it
With deep conviction.

(13)

Blind to *This,* one wanders in Samsara;
Seeing *This,* there is no other Buddha.
In the final Truth, there is neither this, nor that.
May I realize the Dharma-nature—
The meaning and Origin of all!

(14)

Manifestation is mind;
And so is Voidness too.
Enlightenment is mind;
And so is blindness too.
The emergence and extinction
Of things are also in one's mind.
May I understand that all and everything
Inhere only in the mind.

(15)

Unsullied by intended practice and by efforts,
And apart from worldly influence and distractions,
May I rest at ease in mind's natural state
And learn the subtle teaching of Mind-practice.

(16)

Strong and weak, clear and dim,
The waves of flowing thoughts subside.
Without disturbance the mind-river gently flows.
Far from the mud of drowsiness and distractions,
May I enter the steady ocean of Samadhi!

(17)

Often I contemplate the incontemplatable
Mind, clearly I discern Truth indiscernable.
Ever may I eliminate the doubts of "Yes" and "No,"
With certainty may I behold my own Self-face!

(18)

Observing outer objects, I find but my own mind;
Observing my mind, I find only Voidness;
Observing both mind and objects,
I am freed from the Two Clingings.
May I realize the Self-nature of the illuminating mind!

(19)

Because *That* transcends the mind,
It is the Great Symbol called;
Because *That* frees from the extremes,
It is called the Great Middle Way;
Because *That* embraces all,
It is called the Great Perfection;
May I ever understand that knowing one is knowing all.

(20)

Because of no attachment, the Great
Bliss continuously arises.
Free from clinging, the radiant Light
Outshines hindrances and shade.
May I practice without ceasing this Practice-of-no-effort,
Which is free, beyond thought, and self-sustaining.

(21)

The craving for ecstasy and good experience on its
    own dissolves;
Confusions and evil thoughts are self-purified in
    the Dharmadhatu;
The *ordinary mind*⁷ has no acceptance or rejection,
    no loss or gain;
May I ever realize the truth of Dharma-nature —
That which is far beyond all playwords.

(22)

Not knowing that their Self-nature
Is identical with Buddha's,
Sentient beings ever wander in Samsara.
Toward all creatures bound by sorrow
Who suffer infinite pain
May I always have true pity,
Through great, unbearable compassion.

(23)

When this compassion rises, the great Voidness
Also becomes vivid in its nakedness.
This clear and supreme Path that's Two-in-One,
Day and night may I ever follow it.

(24)

May I use clairvoyance and like
Powers gained through meditation,
To ripen sentient beings,
To serve all Buddhas and their Lands.
May I fulfill the great wishes of the Enlightened Ones,
And quickly attain supreme and perfect Buddhahood.

(25)

Great is the power of all virtues in the Universe,
Great is the power of Buddha and Bodhisattvas'
    Compassions.
With the support of this great might,
And guided by the Light of Dharma,
May all my good wishes be fulfilled
Readily, and those of others.

The Essentials
of Mahamudra Practice

As Given by
the Venerable Lama Kong Ka

LAMA KONG KA SAID:

"To practice this Mahamudra meditation one should first be initiated by a qualified Guru. The purpose of Mahamudra initiation is to make the disciple recognize the illuminating-void Awarness of his Self-mind. Only after recognizing this intrinsic 'awareness-without-content' can the disciple practice Mahamudra correctly. Until he has done so, he will find it difficult to escape from the subject-object entanglement and to elevate his mind to the state of non-distinction and non-attachment. To deepen this illuminating-void Awareness, he should practice often the essential instructions given below.

"He who can rest his mind in pure Self-awareness without distraction will be able to do anything. To practice Mahamudra he should stop discriminating, abandon habitual thoughts of 'accept this' and 'reject that,' and strive to reach a state where Samadhi and activities become one. Until he has done so, he should stress quiet meditation first, and then as a subsidiary exercise apply his Mahamudra-awareness to his daily activities."

* * *

"There are three essentials in the Mahamudra practice: *equilibrium, relaxation,* and *naturalness.*

" 'Equilibrium' means to balance body, mouth, and mind.
The Mahamudra way of balancing the body is to loosen
it, of balancing the mouth is to slow down the breathing,
and of balancing the mind is not to cling to and rely on
anything.

"This is the supreme way to tame the body, breath
[prana], and mind.

" 'Relaxation' means to loosen the mind, to let everything
go, to strip off all ideas and thoughts. When one's whole
body and mind become loose, one can, without effort, remain in the natural state, which is intrinsically non-dis-
criminative and yet without distractions.

" 'Naturalness' means not 'taking' or 'leaving' anything:
in other words the yogi does not make the slightest effort
of any kind. He lets the senses and mind stop or flow by
themselves without assisting or restricting them. To practice
naturalness is to make no effort and be spontaneous.

"The above can be summarized thus:

The essence of equilibrium is not to cling.
The essence of relaxation is not to hold.
The essence of naturalness is to make no effort."

THE FIVE SIMILES
OF MAHAMUDRA EXPERIENCE

"There are five similes which describe the correct experience of Mahamudra:

A sphere which is vast like infinite space.
Awareness omnipresent like the great earth.
A mind steady as a mountain.

Self-realizing Awareness clear and bright like
a lamp.
Pure consciousness, crystal clear and empty of
discriminating thoughts.

"Mahamūdra experience can also be described thus:

Like a cloudless sky, the sphere is broad
and free from obstruction.
Like a waveless ocean, the mind is steady
without discriminating thoughts.
Like a bright lamp on a windless night, the
consciousness is clear, bright, and stable."

* * *

"To practice Mahamudra, keep both mind and body
loose and gentle without straining to do so; stop doubting
and worrying, and remain balanced.

"In practicing Mahamudra, identify all that you en-
counter with the 'unborn Void' and remain natural and
relaxed."

* * *

"To keep the body loose and gentle does not imply
completely abandoning all activities, but that these activities
should be carried out in a smooth, relaxed, and spontaneous
way.

"To keep the mind loose and gentle does not imply
making it dumb or insensible, but that one should try to
further and sharpen its bright awareness.

"To identify everything with the Unborn Void means
that he who has realized Self-awareness and is able to sus-

tain it, should then try to let everything he meets and
experiences liberate itself into the Voidness."

THE FIVE WAYS OF STRAYING
FROM MAHAMUDRA

"(1) One is liable to misconstrue Voidness as an annul-
ment of both virtues and vices if he does not know that
existence and Voidness are, in essence, identical, and this
includes all moral truths and laws. This misunderstanding
is straying from the View of Mahamudra. On the other
hand, if one only has some sort of understanding of this
truth, but cannot experience it intimately, he is said to
have strayed from the realization of Mahamudra.

"(2) If one does not know that Mahamudra practice
[the Path] is, in essence, not different from Mahamudra
accomplishment [the Fruit] and that all the wondrous merits
are contained in the practice itself, he is liable to think
that practice comes first and Realization follows, so that
Enlightenment is a product of the practice. This is perhaps
true on the everyday level, but as far as the View is con-
cerned, he is said to have gone astray.

"(3) If one can make a genuine effort in Mahamudra
practice but does not have immutable faith in the teaching
itself, he is liable to cherish a 'hidden' hope that some
day he may attain a teaching that is superior even to Mahamudra. This is also a sign of straying from Mahamudra.

"(4) He who knows not that *the cure* and *the cured*
are, in essence, the same, is liable to cling to the idea that

the Dharma-practice [the cure] and the desire-passions [the cured, or that which is to be cured] are two absolutely different things. This is also straying from the View of Mahamudra.

(5) In Mahamudra practice, there is always a tendency on the yogi's part to make too many corrections. He who finds himself always trying to correct faults is most likely to have strayed from the Path."

THE THREE MAJOR EXPERIENCES
OF MAHAMUDRA

"In the course of meditation practice, three major experiences will be encountered. They are: Blissfulness, Illumination, and Non-distinction.

"(1) In the experience of Blissfulness some people feel that a great rapture envelops the whole body and does not decrease even in adverse circumstances, such as in extremely cold or hot weather. Some may feel that both body and mind disappear, that they are extremely joyful — and they often burst into laughter. Some may feel full of inspiration and enthusiasm, or extremely peaceful, contented, and happy. The ecstasy may become so great and intense that they become unconscious of day and night.

"(2) In the experience of Non-distinction, some may feel that all things become empty, or may see the void nature of the world; others experience all things as devoid of self-entity, or that both body and mind are non-existent; while yet others really understand the truth of Voidness [Sunyata]."

"None of the above experiences should be treated as perfect and complete, and one should never cling to any of them. Among them, that of Non-distinction is most important and unerring. Some of the Illumination and Blissfulness experienced *could* be very misleading and even harmful."

*   *   *

"The profoundest of all the verbal instructions on Mahamudra is this:

Cast aside all clinging and the essence will at once emerge.

"The core of Mahamudra practice consists of two things, non-effort and non-correction. One should know, however, what this non-correction means. The Jetsun Milarepa explained this point very clearly: 'Concerning the practice of non-correction, one should understand three things: If wandering thoughts and desire-passions are not corrected, one will fall into the lower realms. If the Blissfulness, Illumination, and Non-distinction are not corrected, one will fall into the Three Realms of Samsara.[1] Only the immanent Self-mind needs no correction.' "

*   *   *

"At all times in the day, during or after meditation, one should try not to lose the 'essence.' In other words, one should try to bring the meditation experience into his daily activities.

"It is quite understandable that one may be distracted during his daily work, thus forgetting the 'essence,' but he should try always to bring back the Awareness, and if he succeeds, the 'essence' will at once emerge again.

"One should try not to lose Self-awareness by day or night. To practice Mahamudra during sleep and in dreams is also extremely important. He who cannot do so properly should shun all activities and practice Mahamudra meditation uninterruptedly for five or six days, then he should rest for one day before continuing. One should not be discouraged if he cannot keep the Awareness alive for a whole day. To make a continuous and persistent effort is essential. He who can do so will certainly broaden his Awareness and Realization."

HOW TO CULTIVATE MAHAMUDRA THROUGH ADVERSE CONDITIONS

"After one has realized the 'essence,' he should then proceed to practice the so-called 'utilizing exercises.' That is to say one should utilize some particular conditions to further Realization.

"(1) *To utilize distraction and discriminating thoughts to further Realization:*

"This does not mean observing the nature of discriminating thoughts, nor meditating on Voidness, nor being 'mindful' of the distraction, but implies keeping 'bright Awareness'—the essence of discriminating thoughts—vividly alive. This Awareness in its natural state is Mahamudra.

If at first one has great difficulties he should try to over-come them and merge the distracting thoughts into the Path.

"(2) *To utilize desire-passions to further Realization:*

"Sometimes you should purposely stir up desire-passions such as lust, hatred, jealousy, etc.—and then observe them in depth. You should neither follow, relinquish, or correct them but clearly and 'awaringly' remain in a loose and natural state. When in deep sleep you should try to merge Awareness with the unconscious without strain. This is the best way to transform the unconscious into 'light.'

"(3) *To utilize apparitions and devils to further Realization:*

"Whenever any fearful apparition appears, you should employ the Mahamudra meditation on the fears. Do not try to dispel the fear but dwell on it clearly and loosely. In doing so, if the apparition vanishes, you should try once more to conjure up even more frightful apparitions and again apply Mahamudra to them.

"(4) *To utilize compassion and grief to further Realization:*

"Since in the final analysis, life and Samsara imply suffer-ing, a Buddhist should have great compassion for all sentient beings. When contemplating men's sufferings, a great com-passion will arise; right at the very moment when that compassion arises, one should practice the Mahamudra meditation on it. When one does so, both Wisdom and Compassion will grow.

"(5) *To utilize sickness to further Realization:*

"Whenever you are ill, you should practice the Ma-hamudra meditation on the sickness. You should also observe penetratingly the essence both of the patient and of the sickness, thus eliminating the dualism of subject and object.

"(6) *To utilize death to further Realization:*

"He who can practice Mahamudra as instructed will not be perplexed or frightened when death occurs. He will then be able to identify, without fear, all the visions and experiences that take place in the process of dying. Free from attachment and expectations he can then unify the Light of the Mother and Son[2] into one great whole."

THE ERRORS IN MAHAMUDRA PRACTICE

"(1) If one's Mahamudra practice is confined solely to the effort of stabilizing the mind, the activities of all one's six consciousnesses will be halted, or dimmed. This is called a 'frozen ice' type of practice, and is a very harmful tendency in Mahamudra meditation which must be avoided.

"(2) He who neglects the clear 'Awareness' but abides solely in Non-distinction will see or hear nothing when confronted with sights, sounds, smells, and touches. . . . This is an error due to having become sluggish.

"(3) When the last thought has gone, and the next one has not come, this immediate, present moment is a very wonderful thing if one can abide therein; *but,* if he does so without clear awareness, he still falls into the error of sluggishness.

"(4) He who can hold the bright Awareness but thinks there is nothing more to Mahamudra also falls into error.

"(5) If one only cultivates 'Blissfulness,' 'Illumination,' and 'Non-distinction' without practicing 'penetrating-obser-vation-into-the-mind,' it still cannot be considered as the correct Mahamudra practice.

"(6) He who develops a dislike to manifestations is most likely to have gone astray.

"(7) He who concentrates on his Awareness and culti-vates the illuminating-void Self-mind is said to practice Mahamudra correctly. However, this 'concentration-effort' has a tendency to hinder that spontaneity and freedom of spirit, without which it is difficult to unfold the vast and liberating Mind. One should therefore never forget to prac-tice the 'looseness,' 'vastness,' and 'spontaneity.' "

*   *   *

"What, then, is the correct Mahamudra practice?
"[Answer:] The ordinary mind [Tib.: Thal.Ma.Ces.Pa.] is itself the correct practice. That is to say, to let the ordinary mind remain in its own natural state. If to this mind one adds or subtracts anything, it is then not the ordinary mind but the so-called 'mind-object' [Tib.: Yul.]. To make not the slightest intention and effort to practice, and yet not to be distracted for a single moment, is to practice the natural mind correctly. Therefore, as long as you can keep your Self-awareness, no matter what you do, you are still practicing Mahamudra."

NOTES

THE SONG OF MAHĀMUDRĀ

1 *The Song of Mahāmudrā,* known as "Phyg.Chen.Gaṅgā.Ma." in Tibetan, is an important Mahāmudrā text, composed by Tilopa when he imparted this teaching to Nāropa on the bank of the Ganges River.

2 Samaya here implies the Samaya Precepts, i.e., the Precepts a Tantric yogi must observe during his practice. They include fourteen basic Commandments and eighty subsidiary Rules.

3 Ālaya: the Ālaya Consciousness. (For a definition, see the Glossary.)

4 Dharmatā: the essence or nature of the Dharma; the nature underlying all things, reality, and the like.

5 The Mother- and Son-Light (T.T.: Mahi.Hod.Zer. [and] Buhi.-Hod.Zer.): The Mother-Light, the innate Light or Dharmakāya, exists within oneself at all times, but the uninitiated cannot realize it. The Son-Light is not a different light outside of the Mother-Light, but the *realization* of the Mother-Light in the Path. The reasons for the nomenclature "Son-Light" are because, (1) without the innate Mother-Light no Realization is possible, as without a mother there will be no son, and (2) the Mother-Light is always complete, perfect, and changeless, whereas the Son-Light can be varied at different times in the Path.

THE VOW OF MAHĀMUDRĀ

1 The text of *The Vow of Mahāmudrā* (T.T.: Phyag.Chen.sMon.-Lam.) is used as a daily prayer by the Ghagyuba Lamas. It was written by Garmapa Raṅ.Byuṅ.rDo.rJe. (A.D. 1284-1339).

.

2 The Four Bodies of Buddha: the Transformation Body (T.T.: sPrul.sKu.), the Reward Body (T.T.: Loñs.sPyod.rDsogs.Pahi.-sKu.), the Dharma Body (T.T.; Chos.sKu.), and the Body of Universal Essence (T.T.: Chos.dByiñs.Ño.Bo.Ñid.Gyi.sKu.).

3 The Holy and Rational Judgments (T.T.: Luñ. [and] Rigs.Pa.): two sure ways to find the Truth, i.e., by depending on the holy Scriptures and by correct and logical reasoning.

4 Two Truths: the Mundane Truth (T.T.: Kun.rDsob.bDen.Pa.), and the Transcendental Truth (T.T.: Don.Dam.bDen.Pa.).

5 Two Benefits (T.T.: Don.gÑis.): the conduct that contributes either to the benefit of self or to that of others.

6 Two Clingings (T.T.: hDsin.gÑis.): the clinging to the inner self and the clinging to outer objects.

THE ESSENTIALS OF MAHĀMUDRĀ PRACTICE

1 Three Realms: the Realms of Desire (T.T.: hDod.Khams.), of Form (T.T.: gZugs.Khams.), and of Formlessness (T.T.: gZugs.-Med.Khams.). These include all the three major types of sentient beings in the Three Realms of Saṃsāra. Sentient beings in the Realm of Desire all have strong desire-passions (kleśas); in the Realm of Form they have fewer desire-passions; and in the Realm of Formlessness still fewer. The Realms of Form and Formlessness consist of the so-called Twenty-four Heavens. To be born there, one must attain the various Dhyānas or Samādhis; but all these Heavens and Dhyānas, according to Buddhism, are still Saṃsāric, and they alone cannot lead one to Liberation. According to Mahāmudrā, those who cling to the Blissfulness of Samādhi will be born in the Heaven of Desire; those to Illumination, will be born in the Heaven of Form; and those to Non-distinction, will be born in the Heaven of Formlessness.

2 See Note 5 under *The Song of Mahāmudrā.*

Part II

The Epitome of
an Introduction to the
Six Yogas of Naropa

The Epitome of
an Introduction to the
Profound Path of the
Six Yogas of Naropa

by
Drashi Namjhal

OBEISANCE TO GURU DORJE-CHANG.

The identity of noumenon and phenomenon
Is the reality of Dharma.
The oneness of Skill and Wisdom
Is the Path of the Bliss-Void.
The sameness of forms and the Void
Is the Fruit of the Trikaya.[1]
To Vajradhara[2] who shows
The Path, I make obeisance.

Composing body, mouth, and mind
He mastered the three Yogas,[3]
Earning the Supreme Accomplishment;[4]
To Gambopa,[5] peerless Guru,
I make my sincere obeisance.

The blissful Void of Dumo Heat[6]
Is the essence of magic play.
The Yogas of the Illusory-Body
And of Dream are of Light the essence.

In the Bardo[7] realm, to win Trikaya
Excels the birth in Buddha's Paradise.
To Gurus in the Lineage
Who have mastered all these Yogas,
I make my sincere obeisance.

The Pith-Instructions[8] of these Six Yogas[9]
Are here set forth to help the capable.
O, Lord of Secrets[10] and of Dakinis,[11]
I beg Thee to guide us with Thy blessing.

This Teaching is given for those who have renounced the
world, and aspire to attain Buddhahood in this very life.
It is to assist those capable devotees of the Two Yogas[12]
speedily to attain the Trikaya of Buddhahood, that this
explanation of the quintessential Teachings of the Profound
Path is written.

First, we shall briefly review the underlying principles
of the practice [of the Six Yogas]; then we shall discuss
the various practices in detail; and finally we shall comment
briefly on the result, or Accomplishment.

The Basic Principles of Tantric Practice

The basic principles of this [Tantric] practice lie in an
understanding of [the correspondence between the human
body and the Body of Buddhahood]. Therefore, one should
understand the nature of the energies [pranas], psychic-
nerves [nadis], and secretions [bindus], and the over-all

functions of the physical body. Generally speaking, the yogi should know the construction of the Vajra Body, made of the Six Elements[13]—its creation, existence, and decay. Specifically, he should know how the nadis, pranas, and bindus function, and thoroughly understand the mind's nature and the various forms that it can take. He should also know that all things are projected by the Alaya Consciousness[14] in its crude, subtle, and most subtle manifestations. The crude manifestation implies the totality of the Seven Consciousnesses,[15] the subtle indicates the eighty types of distracting thoughts,[16] and the most subtle denotes the stages of "Revelation," "Augmentation," and "Attainment."[17] One should also be familiar with the theory of how and why these three phenomena take place and pass away. In addition, one should become well acquainted with the basic principles of the Foundation, Path, and Accomplishment of Tantrism:[18] the passion-desires that must be transformed, the Path to be followed, and the great Wisdom to be attained. All these points should be studied carefully in the different Scriptures, and contemplated upon deeply.

THE PRACTICE OF THE SIX YOGAS

Before one engages in the main practice of the Six Yogas, some preliminaries are required. These include basic meditations on the transiency of life, on the sufferings of Samsara, on the difficulty of obtaining a favorable birth in which to practice the Dharma, on resolute renunciation of this life, on kindness and compassion toward all men, and on the infinite Bodhi-Mind—that great View and vow to bring all sentient beings to the state of Buddhahood. Only through these practices can the foundation of Dharma be built. The yogi should then proceed to practice the Tantric preliminaries as follows:

To purify worldly clingings and to lay a good foundation for the advanced practice of the Six Yogas, the disciple should first obtain the four complete Initiations of Dem-chog,[19] and practice the Arising Yoga[20] until he has reached a fairly stabilized stage. To conquer inertia and laziness, he should meditate more on death; to overcome his hindrances, he should pray to the Buddhas and arouse the Bodhi-Mind; to prepare sufficient provisions for the Path of Dharma, he should give alms and make the Mandala offerings; to cleanse himself from sins and transgressions, he should repent and recite the Mantra of Vajrasattva; to attain the Blessings, he should practice the Guru Yoga. Each of these preparatory practices can be carried out in five to seven consecutive days. Their instructions and rituals are available in other sources.

The main practice of the Six Yogas is set forth as follows:

1. Instructions on the Heat, or Dumo Yoga—the Foundation of the Path.
2. Instructions on the Illusory-Body Yoga—the Reliance of the Path.
3. Instructions on the Dream Yoga—the Yardstick of the Path.
4. Instructions on the Light Yoga—the Essence of the Path.
5. Instructions on the Bardo Yoga—that which is met on the Path.
6. Instructions on the Transformation Yoga—the Core of the Path.

1. INSTRUCTIONS ON THE HEAT, OR DUMO YOGA

A. THE ELEMENTARY PRACTICE

The elementary practice of Heat Yoga has five successive steps:

(1) Visualizing the Emptiness, or Hollowness of the Body.
(2) Visualizing the Main Psychic-Nerves, or Nadis.
(3) [Vase-] Breathing Exercises.
(4) Manipulating the Bindus.
(5) Bodily Exercises.

(1) Visualizing the Emptiness, or Hollowness of the Body

At first the yogi should pray to his Guru for a steady growth of Dumo Heat. He should sit in the "Seven-fold seated posture of Buddha Vairocana": Cross the legs in the Lotus Posture; place both hands, one upon the other, below the navel; straighten the spine like an arrow; slightly bend the neck to press the throat; place the tongue against the roof of the mouth; and focus the eyes upon the tip of the nose. Then the yogi should visualize his body as becoming that of the Patron Buddha—but empty within like a balloon. From the head down to the tips of the toes there is only hollowness. If he cannot see the whole body as completely hollow he should try to visualize a part at a time. For instance, he can visualize the hollowness of the head, of the neck, of the arms, of the chest, and the like, until the complete hollowness becomes clear. Then the yogi should visualize his body in different sizes—small as a mustard seed, or large as the whole Universe, but all hollow within. He should practice this with great diligence until the vision of the hollow body becomes extremely clear.

(2) Visualizing the Main Psychic-Nerves, or Nadis

When the vision of body-hollowness has become clear, the yogi should then visualize the Central Channel in the center of the body. Its upper end reaches the top of the head, and then curves down to the point between the two eyebrows; its lower end reaches a point about four fingers below the navel; its width is that of whipcord; and its color is white on the outside and red within. The yogi should also visualize the other two Channels, namely, the Right and Left [Roma and Junma]. Their width is that of an arrow shaft; the color of the Right Channel is red slightly tinged with white, and that of the Left, vice versa. These two Channels run parallel to but about half an inch from the Central one. Their upper ends also reach the top of the head and then curve down to the two nostrils. All three Channels are hollow, straight, clear, and transparent. Some instructions say that the Central Channel is as thick as an arrow shaft and the other two as thick as [wheat] stalks; that the Right and Left Channels should be visualized as the intestines of a goat—hoary and old; that the Central Channel should be visualized as blue in color, the Right is red, and the Left as white; others say that all three Channels are white on the outside and red inside. Although these instructions vary in many ways, one can choose any one of them for practice.

Some instructions add that the upper end of the Central Channel reaches the Gate of Purity[21] and the lower end extends all the way down to the opening in the privy organ. But I think it would be better to follow the instructions given above.

When these three Channels[22] are seen clearly, the yogi should then visualize the Four Cakras[23] in the head, throat,

chest, and navel, respectively. The Navel Cakra is also
called the Transformation Center, and has sixty-four nadis
extending upward like the ribs of a reversed unbrella; the
Heart Cakra is called the Dharma Center, with eight nadis
extending downward like an umbrella's ribs; the Throat
Cakra is called the Enjoyment Center, with sixteen nadis
extending upward; and the Head Cakra, the Great Joy
Center, has thirty-two nadis extending downward. All four
Cakras are connected with, or "sprout" from the Central
Channel, as ribs from the stick of an umbrella. From the
tip of each nadi numerous thin "nerves" spread out to cover
all parts of the body—forming innumerable networks or
plexus. All these nadis are red inside and white outside,
and each is hollow within. Some say that they are either
red or yellow, some that the Throat and Navel Centers are
red, the Heart Center white, and the Head Center green.
One may, however, practice either way. If one cannot visualize them clearly all at once, he should visualize a part at
a time. But the important point is to make the vision extremely clear, [especially that of the three main nadis, or
Channels, and the Four Cakras]. Some instructions say
that in addition to these four Cakras, the Crown Cakra and
the Privy Cakra should be added, thus making a total of
six; some say one may visualize all the 72,000 nadis in the
entire body. But I think one can do with, or without, these
additional Cakras and nadis.

(3) The Vase-Breathing Exercises

The best time to practice Vase-Breathing is when the
breath flows evenly through both nostrils. If one finds that
more air is passing through one nostril than the other, he
should lie down on that side and use the thumb to close

that nostril, forcing the air out through the other one. After a number of breaths, he will find the air running evenly through both nostrils.

Now sit up, use a finger to close the left nostril, and make a long exhalation through the right one. Then, [after inhaling] make a short exhalation, then a long and gentle one. Practice this three times, then do the same with the left nostril, and finally with both nostrils.

When breathing out, the Yogi should think that all hindrances, sins, and sicknesses in the body are expelled. Those who have never practiced this exercise before should press each nostril with the index finger of the same side, and press the side of the chest with the opposite arm and fist when breathing out. The yogi should put his two fists on both knees when breathing through both nostrils. After each exhalation he should inhale deeply, bending the neck slightly before he breathes out again. This is called the "Breath of Nine Blowings," and should only be done once or twice at the outset of meditation. If one practices it too much, he will have headaches and breathing troubles. But sometimes, in the middle of a meditation, he can practice this exercises very gently when needed.

Now, the main practice of the Vase-Breathing exercise:

Sit as instructed before, and straighten the spine slightly. Put a pillow or blanket about three inches thick under the hips. Then draw in gently a long, subtle breath, pressing the air down below the navel, and swallow spittle with the air. Now contract the sphincter muscle of the anus slightly, and hold the air at the Navel Cakra.

When the yogi has become proficient in pressing down the air, he can then contract the sphincter muscle more strongly than before without moving the abdomen. This practice—of pressing the upper air down, pulling the lower air up, and mingling them at the Navel Center so that the protruding lower belly takes the shape of a vase or pot—is, for this reason, called the "Vase-Breathing Exercise."

When the yogi can hold the air no longer, he should take a very short breath to relieve the tension, roll the belly muscle three times, and try to hold the breath once more as long as possible. When he can do so no longer, he should raise the head slightly and release the air as slowly as he can. These four processes are called *inhaling, filling, dissolving,* and *shooting.*

Some visualizations should be practiced during the Vase-Breathing exercise. When *inhaling,* visualize the pranas of the Five Elements, in five different colors, being drawn into the nostrils from a distance of about ten inches from the nose; when *filling,* visualize the air descending through both Channels as though inflating the intestines of a goat, passing through the intersection point, entering the Central Channel, and remaining there; when *dissolving,* visualize the air circulating [within] the Central Channel; when *shooting,* visualize a Tig Le,[24] which symbolizes the Essence of Prana-Mind,[25] shooting up through the Central Channel and out at the Head Center. This *shooting* visualization, however, should only be practiced once at the start of a meditation; to do so too often leads to trouble.

According to some Gurus, during the shooting process one should imagine the air leaving the body through the midpoint between the two eyebrows. According to another instruction, the pranas of the Five Elements should be visualized as Five-colored light-beams emanating from numerous tiny triangular-shaped thunderbolts [dorjes].

These tiny dorjes enter, emerge, and remain in the body during the *inhaling, exhaling,* and *holding* process, respectively. Some say that during the *dissolving* process one should first visualize the air as filling the Central Channel, then the Four Cakras, and finally all the nadis of the entire body; but this is criticized by others as a bad method which will cause air to leak from the body.

It is never advisable to start with this intensive type of Vase-Breathing, because while one may gain some temporary experiences, he will not benefit much in the long run; besides, he will meet with innumerable [other] difficulties. Therefore a beginner is not advised to practice the vigorous type of Vase-Breathing; instead, he should practice the gentle Vase-Breathing, which will do him a world of good with little or no hindrances. Also, he is strongly recommended not to practice any vigorous type of Vase-Breathing before he has become proficient with the gentle one. The so-called gentle Vase-Breathing is to hold the air for a short while, release it before there is any strain, then at once draw in another breath and hold it again. All this should be repeated eight to ten times, making one complete round. Then the yogi may rest for a short while before repeating it. One should try to prolong the holding period gradually and gently; he should never breathe through the mouth, and should avoid any place where the air is smoky or bad while doing this exercise.

If one can hold the breath without strain for two minutes, he is considered to have fulfilled the minimum requirement for mastering the pranas; for four minutes is average; but if for six minutes or more, that is the highest requirement.

Here a few words should be said about the [preliminary] sign of the pranas entering the Central Channel. This takes place when, at any time during meditation, the breath begins to flow smoothly and evenly through both nostrils, then becomes extremely subtle, and finally stops completely. This phenomenon, however, can also occur when the prana sinks or leaks [?]. If the former, one feels his mind becoming dim and sluggish; if the latter, he cannot visualize at all clearly. But these phenomena do not happen in the case of the pranas' entering the Central Channel. One should bear this great difference in mind.

(4) Manipulating the Bindus

The yogi should visualize a small white drop [like a dewdrop], about the size of a small pea, sparkling but transparent, at the midpoint between his eyebrows. He should think that this drop [Tig Le, or bindu] is the embodiment of his own mind, and visualize it until it becomes extremely clear. Then, while breathing in as above, he should visualize the Tig Le ascending from between the eyebrows to the upper end of the Central Channel; and during the *holding* process, he should concentrate on it. While he breathes out he should imagine the Tig Le flowing down again to the midpoint between the brows. He should do all this several times. Then, he takes a long breath and pushes the air down to the Navel Center. At the same time he should imagine that the Tig Le drops down to the Navel Center through the Central Channel like a small iron ball falling through a tube with a rattle; then, while holding the breath, he should concentrate on the Tig Le at the Navel Center. When he exhales, the Tig Le returns again to the Head Center through the Central Channel.

[Steadily to improve this meditation] the yogi should first visualize the Tig Le dropping down only to the Throat

Center until, without effort, the vision becomes extremely clear. Finally he should visualize the Tig Le dropping down first to the Heart and then to the Navel Center.

After mastering this practice, the Yogi should concentrate upon the Tig Le at a given Cakra [especially the Navel Cakra] and at the same time practice the Vase-Breathing five to seven times. One should notice here that during inhalation, the Tig Le drops down to the lower Cakras; when the breath is held, it remains in the center of the Cakra; and during exhalation, it returns to the midpoint between the eyebrows. At the end of every meditation one should concentrate upon this Center.

(5) Bodily Exercises

It is through bodily exercises that many of the knots in the nadis are untied. They improve the flow of the pranas and Tig Les in the nadis; they also rejuvenate impaired pranas, nadis, and Tig Les. One should therefore learn and practice the various bodily exercises given in Tantric texts; this is extremely important. Special attention should be paid to the practice of the Six Rotation Exercises of Naropa —a fundamental exercise of the Heat Yoga—both at the beginning and end of meditation. He should also practice for specific purposes other exercises which he can find in my volume, *The Red Book of Heat Yoga*. [This book is unavailable at the present time, either in Tibetan, or in English translation. Tr.]

Now, to build a good foundation for Heat Yoga, the following practices should be stressed:

Sit on the floor, cross the legs, put a high pillow under the hips, and tie a cotton belt to fasten the waist and knees to steady the body during meditation.

Sitting in the "Seven-fold Seated Posture of Vairocana" as instructed before, the yogi may now practice the Vase-Breathing exercise, but he should not do so when too full or too hungry, nor at noon or midnight. The best time is when the breath flows evenly through both nostrils.[26] One should therefore start to practice when the breathing is about to shift from one nostril to the other, for then the breath is balanced in both nostrils. When visualizing, this does not alter the effort made on the nadis, but more stress should be placed on seeing the Dumo-fire at the intersection of the Three Channels below the navel. This Dumo-fire is shaped like a small Tibetan *A* [ཨ] word [or an ovoid or almond-shaped flame with a sharp and narrow tongue which tapers to a point like a twisted needle or a thin cork-screw]. Reddish-brown, intensely hot and undulating, it can produce heat and bliss in all nadis throughout the body.

When *inhaling* and *filling*, the yogi should imagine the air flowing down the Right and Left Channels, and, like the wind from a bellows, fanning the Dumo-fire to an intense heat; when *dissolving,* he should think of all the pranas in the body as gathering at, and evaporating into, this Dumo-fire. During the ["shooting" or] exhalation, the Dumo rises through the Central Channel.

The fire of Dumo is the foundation of Heat Yoga; it should therefore be visualized very clearly in order actually to produce heat. A firm and clear visualization of the Dumo must be established [before one can hope for substantial progress]. At the start, the blazing tongue of Dumo should not be visualized as more than the height of a finger's breadth; then gradually it increases in height to two, three, and four fingers' breadth. This blazing tongue of Dumo is thin and long, shaped like a twisted needle or the long

hair of a hog; it also possesses all four characteristics of
the Four Elements—the firmness of earth, the wetness of
water, the warmth of fire, and the mobility of air; but its
outstanding quality still lies in its great heat—which can
evaporate the pranas and produce the Bliss.

The yogi who follows the above instructions should be
able to lay a good foundation for Dumo Yoga and produce
the Heat and Bliss.

Some say that in the Heat Yoga practice one should
also visualize the four bija syllables[27] in the Four Cakras.
This is described in the *Tantras of Hevajra* and *Demchog,*
but not in most writings of the Six Yogas.

B. THE MORE ADVANCED PRACTICE

The above instructions were all directed toward the
elementary or basic practice. We shall now deal with the
more advanced practice, with specific emphasis on:

(1) How to increase the Dumo, or Heat
(2) How to increase the Bliss
(3) How to increase the Non-distinction
(4) How to improve the Bliss-Void Samadhi
(5) How to conquer the hindrances in Dumo practice

(1) How to Increase the Dumo, or Heat

In order to increase the Heat, the yogi may lengthen the
tongue of Dumo-fire up to eight fingers' breadth, but he
should still concentrate mainly on the original Dumo itself
—the source from which the fire-tongue springs. He may
then visualize the tongue of fire rising to the Heart, Throat,
or even the Head Center. Some say that the Dumo should
not be visualized above the Throat Center, but since what

concerns us here is the production of more heat, it is correct to do so. The yogi may also think of the Dumo-fire spreading into all the nadis—large or small, long or short—throughout the entire body. Thus the whole body becomes a blazing fireball. At the end of this meditation, all the fire should be withdrawn to the main Dumo.

If, in following this practice, one still cannot produce the Heat, or can produce it only in one part of the body, he may try the following exercise:

Sit with the legs crossed and arms wrapped around the knees; then hold the Vase-Breath, while rotating the lower part of the abdomen clockwise and counterclockwise many times; protrude and retract the abdomen many times; massage the body, especially the colder parts; . . . and also perform other bodily exercises to increase the Heat. All these should be done while holding the breath. To visualize a great fire raging throughout the body will also help to increase the Heat, but the most important thing is still to think of the Dumo-fire as blazing within the Central Channel. . . .

Although the vigorous exercises, such as strong Vase-Breathing, bodily movements, etc., can generate heat quickly, the heat so produced is not steady, and cannot last very long. The benefit, therefore, is very small. But if one can produce Dumo-heat gradually and steadily, that heat will not lessen, and immeasurable benefit will be gained.

Even when it is bitterly cold, the yogi should not wear fur garments; and when it is very hot he should never go naked. Nor should he get close to a fire, expose himself to the hot sun, blow a large trumpet, or breathe through the mouth. He should practice the "Ever-stable Vase-Breathing"[28] at all times, eat good and nourishing food, and carefully guard his Tig Le.

If intensive heat is generated in a certain part of the body, throughout it, or between flesh and skin, the yogi should know that this is a symptom of the sudden kindling of the Fire-prana. But as this heat is not stable and will soon disappear, he should pay no attention to it but concentrate on the Dumo in the Navel Center, and try to lead the pranas into the Central Channel.

If he feels a blissful or "ecstatic" heat in the Navel Center, while it gradually increases and begins to spread throughout the body, he should know that this is the genuine Dumo-heat which increases greatly the production of the red and white Tig Les.

If the yogi follows these instructions but still cannot produce the Dumo, he should do more bodily exercises, such as the "Six Body Movements of Naropa," and so on, as given elsewhere. [See pp. 62, 63. Further exposition is not given in this book. Tr.]

(2) How to Increase the Bliss

Sit on the ground, with the heel of the left foot [pressed into the groin] close under the sphincter muscle of the anus [to prevent the leakage of Tig Le]. Then visualize the white Tig Le embodied in the reversed Tibetan syllable *Ham* [𑖠]—the size of a pea, snow-white in color, round in shape, sparkling with radiance, and situated in the Head Center. Also visualize the Dumo-fire in the Navel Center— its upper end thin as a needle but intensely hot—which begins to generate penetrating heat within the Central Channel; as a result, the white Tig Le of the Head Center begins to melt and drip down. Through this melting of the Tig Le a great Bliss is produced. In this bliss-producing practice the yogi should inhale air to fan the Dumo-heat below the Navel, which in turn continues to melt the white Tig Le at the Head Center, causing it to drip down incessantly [and inexhaustibly] to the Throat Center and spread through all the nadis thereof. A great bliss and heat, permeating the entire body, is thus generated. Then the flow of the dripping Tig Le spreads down to the Navel Center, in turn producing even greater bliss. . . .

If this visualization can only produce a slight bliss, the following practice should be stressed:

Think that the Dumo-fire, thin as a needle, lengthens upward from the Navel to the Head Center, touching the white Tig Le, melting it, and causing it to spread through the nadis of the Head Center; at the same time imagine that even more bliss is produced; then concentrate on this blissful experience for a short time. In this manner the yogi should visualize the Tig Le dripping down and spreading through all Four Cakras.

After this, the "reversing exercise" should be applied by visualizing the white Tig Le's return to the Head Center. Both the descending and ascending of the Tig Le should be frequently practiced. In addition, the yogi should visualize the white Tig Le and Dumo as merging into one and spreading over the entire body through the innumerable nadis, thus producing great bliss. When the dripping white Tig Le descends upon the Dumo-fire, the latter shrinks to its original size; and when the white Tig Le ascends, the Dumo also follows it up to the Head Center.

In the process of *dissolving,* and exhalation, the spine should be kept erect and the merged Tig Les should be spread over the whole body by appropriate bodily movements.

If, in practicing thus, the Bliss still cannot be produced, the yogi should then visualize the lower part of the Central Channel—extending right down to the privy organ—and meditate on the Great Bliss Cakra and its thirty-two nadis. Next he visualizes the white Tig Le continuously dripping down to the organ and spreading through its nadis, and as a result a great bliss is produced. Additional reversing exercises to pull up the Tig Le to the higher Cakras should then be applied. . . .

If these measures still fail to produce a Great Bliss, one may apply the *Wisdom-Mother Mudra* by visualizing the sexual act with a Dakini, while using the breathing to incite the Dumo-heat, to melt the white Tig Le, and so forth. In routine practice the Four Cakras are used; only on the occasion of increasing the Bliss should the Cakra of Great Bliss [the Privy Center] be added and the Wisdom-Mother Mudra applied. If by so doing the yogi cannot hold the Tig Le, he should vigorously pull up the lower pranas, contract the sphincter muscle at the anus, visualize the Tig Le ascending to the Head Center . . . and take other reversing steps. . . . After this, he should at once practice the appropriate bodily exercises a few times to spread the Tig Le throughout the body, and then meditate on the Illuminating Mind-Essence for some time.

Some comments on the experience of Bliss are now needed.

Generally speaking, the Bliss experience can be divided into four categories:

  (a) If the yogi feels his whole body becoming soft and smooth, and experiences a sensation of delight and comfort when he touches anything, this shows that he has "tamed" many nadis in the body. This kind of bliss is therefore called a Nadi-Bliss.

(b) If a sensation of delicate pleasure is felt in a certain part of the body—as when an itch is being scratched —but the sensation is only momentary and soon disappears, the yogi is said to have experienced the Prana-Bliss.

(c) If a feeling of warmth and ecstasy simultaneously arises over the entire body, or in a certain part, this is a bliss produced by increasing the red Tig Le.

(d) If the sensation of bliss is "lustful" like that of the sexual act—intensive and permeating the whole body —it is a bliss produced by the Dumo-fire melting the Tig Le and, according to its intensity, it can be differentiated into three groups:

   (i) If the bliss and lust are so intense and hard to bear that one finds it very difficult to retain the Tig Le, it is then called the "Male Bliss."

   (ii) If the bliss and lust are intensive, but not so strong as the above, and the yogi finds it a little easier to control the Tig Le, it is then considered as the "Female Bliss."

   (iii) If the bliss and lust are not as strong as the above, and the yogi finds it quite easy to control the Tig Le, it is then called the "Neuter Bliss."

One must bear in mind that though these blisses are all due to the Dumo-fire melting the Tig Le, they are not the Great Bliss produced when the pranas enter and dissolve in the Central Channel, which we shall discuss in detail later.

Since the retention of the Tig Le during the experience of ecstasy is of vital importance, some comment should be made here. Generally speaking, most people can usually retain the Tig Le if they can visualize clearly the Three Nadis and Four Cakras with the assistance of some exercises such as the Six Movements of Naropa, and so forth. But there are individuals whose Tig Les are very volatile and difficult to control, so that when they practice the bliss-increasing exercises they find it hard to retain the flow of Tig Le. In this case some special exercises for controlling it, such as the "Bodily Movements of the Tiger," "Elephant," "Turtle," and "Lion" should be practiced, for these are exercises through which the Tig Le can be held, pulled back, and spread. . . .

(3) How to Increase the Non-distinction

According to the Gurus, to further the experience of Non-distinction the yogi should observe with great care the nature of the Bliss produced by Dumo, and also the nature of the mind and its manifestations. He should try to see the void nature of all things and remain in the primordial state as long as he can. In practicing the Yoga of Bliss, he should try to merge the Bliss with Sunyata [Voidness]. This is the general principle of the Non-distinction practice. To those who have already realized Sunyata and the Mind-Essence, these few words will be quite sufficient, but not for those who have not done so, for whom the following is added:

To gain further insight into Non-distinction, the yogi should devote to it half to two thirds of each meditation period. He should not visualize the nadis or Tig Les, nor do any Vase-Breathing exercises or the like, but concentrate on the observation of Voidness. If he has already gained some stability in Samadhi, he should apply its power to further his Sunyata observation; if not, he should first try to attain a stable Samadhi through pranayama [exercise for breath control], or other measures; because unless his Samadhi is stable he cannot observe the Self-mind efficiently and reach the state of Non-distinction. After this, the yogi should apply the "sudden-loose-and-sudden-alert" method to reach the Samadhi that is beyond form, and thereby observe more deeply than before the mind's nature and play. He will then realize that the incomprehensible Mind-Essence is an Illuminating-Void Whole, transcending all conceptualizations, and that all manifestations and wavering thoughts *themselves* are empty, so freeing himself forever from all doubts and fears. The yogi should also observe how the mind arises, remains, and passes away, and try to *feel* these processes in a most intimate manner. The practice of identifying the Void with sound, with manifestation, and with Illumination will also be extremely helpful.

One third of each meditation period should be given to practicing the "soft type" of Vase-Breathing, and the Mahamudra. After meditation one should still try to keep the Awareness alive, and identify all experiences with the Path. For details of this practice, see my *Comprehensive Survey of Mahamudra Meditation.*[29]

(4) How to Improve the Bliss-Void Samadhi

Now I shall comment briefly on how to improve the Bliss-Void Samadhi:

To practice this Samadhi [of the Perfecting Yoga] is to merge one's realization of Sunyata with the Four Blisses produced by Dumo. To practice with the pranas, nadis, and Tig Les, while absorbing one's mind in the Bliss-Void experience, is the most rapid way to Liberation and Enlightenment. But first one must induce a steady Bliss in order to taste, observe, and identify it with Sunyata in the most intimate way. For example, when the melting Tig Le spreads through the Head Cakra, the First Bliss will arise. At this time the yogi should throw his mind right into this Bliss — merging it with the self-illuminating Voidness, or the so-called "Two-in-One Bliss-Void Mahamudra Experience," without the slightest distraction. Practicing thus, the majority of the *crude* forms of distracting thoughts will be subdued. When the Tig Le drops down to the Throat Center and spreads through it, the Supreme Bliss will emerge; and if the yogi then concentrates on the Throat Center while absorbed in the Bliss-Void Samadhi, most of the *subtle* distracting thoughts will be subdued. When the Tig Le descends to the Heart Center and spreads through it, the Third, or the Beyond-Bliss will arise; the yogi should then concentrate on the Heart Center in the Bliss-Void Samadhi, and thus *all* distracting thoughts will be subdued. When the Tig Le drops down to the Navel Cakra . . . the Innate-Born Bliss will arise . . . .

The above process is the so-called Down-coming [or descending] process. After this, the yogi should practice the Up-going [or ascending] process, which is a reversal of the former one . . . . From the Navel, the Tig Le rises to the Heart, Throat, and Head Centers, and the Great Innate-Born Bliss will then arise . . . .

At the end of this meditation, the yogi should disregard all nadis and Cakras, and practice the soft type of Vase-Breathing a number of times, concentrating on Mahamudra and the Dumo. In daily activities, he should also try to retain some sensation of the Bliss-Void experience and should utilize all that he meets with to further this end.

If one concentrates on a Cakra, the pranas will automatically gather there. If the pranas can be concentrated in the Cakras, the Tig Le will also become stabilized, and the Four Bliss-Wisdoms[30] will emerge.

An extremely important point should be clarified here. These Blisses produced when the Tig Le is melted by the Dumo-heat can only induce the "Corresponding," but not the "Actual" Four Bliss-Wisdoms. But whoever through continual practice maintains and stabilizes these Bliss-Void experiences will eventually lead the pranas into the Central Channel . . . and the "Actual" Four Blisses will then emerge. If the yogi can recognize them, and identify them with the illuminating-void Mind-Essence, the Four Bliss-Wisdoms will then arise.

The "Corresponding" Wisdom, which is still tinged with subtle subject-object, or dualistic ideas, is that which unfolds in the initial stage of Sunyata observation. The Real Wisdom is the true Wisdom free from all dualism . . . .

The Four Blisses produced by the Dumo Yoga practice are so vast, and so deep in scope and intensity, that no words can describe them. When one reaches this state he is said to have attained the Bliss-Void Samadhi. Dumo is therefore the foundation of all Tantric practices. The word "Dumo" [T. T.: gTum.Mo.] means "a fierce woman who can destroy all desires and passions"; also, it can be understood as meaning "one who can produce the illuminating-void Wisdom." Dumo is therefore the Fire of Transcendental Wisdom that burns up all ignorance and vice.

The Yogi should also know the four varieties of Dumo:

(a) *Outer Dumo:* the Dumo of the Arising Yoga that can destroy all evils and hindrances.

(b) *Inner Dumo:* the Dumo of Life-Prana that can cure four hundred and four kinds of illness.

(c) *Secret Dumo:* the Dumo of melting and descending that can destroy all desire-passions.

(d) *Transcendental Dumo:* the Dumo of Non-distinction that can bring forth the Innate-Born Wisdom.

(5) How to Conquer the Hindrances in Dumo Practice

The main hindrances to the practice of Dumo Yoga are the four general ones shared by all yogis and devotees — sickness, interruption, desire-passions, and death. But one should not yield to their grip, but fight on with great courage and perseverance. The special difficulties to be met with in Dumo practice are as follows:

In the initial stage, when the nadis in the body are not yet tamed, the yogi will have many *physical* difficulties. He will be harassed by various kinds of sickness and pain, lose strength, or feel very weak. If he has some chronic disease or "old illness," it will now develop. Because the pranas have not yet been tamed in the beginning stage, one encounters [other] weaknesses, and difficulties in holding the breath. Because the Tig Les have not yet spread through the entire body, one's mind cannot function clearly, and thus his experience will be meager. Because the concentration is not yet stable, many distracting thoughts will arise and, as a result, one becomes confused as to right practice and right thinking. Furthermore, if one does not know the correct way to practice, great prana-, nadi-, and bindu-hindrances will occur. All these harassments will impede the yogi's Dumo practice. The cure is simple: courage and perseverance. At this time the yogi should meditate on the sufferings of Samsara, the transiency of life, etc., to arouse a deep sprit of renunciation. He should refresh his aspiration to attain the Two-in-One Vajra Body of Buddhahood, being determined to undergo all pains and trails without a thought of withdrawal. He should also read the biographies of the accomplished Gurus and Sages to strengthen his courage and determination. He should be confident that courage and perseverance can conquer all difficulties in the Path.

On the other hand, if the yogi lives too austerely, he will not have the strength to sustain the Dumo practice. As a result he will be reluctant to practice further, and will stop at the half-way mark. If this has been the case, he should rest thoroughly and eat good and nourishing food to restore his strength and health.

During Dumo practice, if one has tamed the pranas and nadis, he will feel his whole body becoming very smooth and soft; great warmth will be generated [from the Navel Center], and the Tig Le will become volatile and restless . . . . All this makes him feel very blissful and vigorous. But the result is greatly to increase the Tig Les, and lust will grow in proportion. At this crucial time one should be extremely careful and industrious in preserving his Tig Le. If one neglects or relaxes his effort, he will be exposed to the danger of losing the Tig Le — which can happen in the stages of dream, of meditation, and even while awake. The loss of Tig Le is a fatal blow to Dumo Yoga; one should therefore be extremely diligent in preserving it. He should observe the precepts strictly and meditate on the impurities of the human body, and so forth, to subdue the lust. Penetratingly to observe the nature of lust will also help in its conquest.

Generally speaking, the loss of Tig Le harms all meditation practices, but it is always fatal to the Dumo Yoga. No benefit whatsoever can be gained from any form of meditation if one loses his Tig Le. All efforts should therefore be made to preserve this vital force, including the application of further special exercises designed to retain and stabilize it.

When a yogi has made some progress in Dumo practice and gained some good experience of Bliss, Illumination, and Non-distinction, as well as other merits, [he will have a strong urge] to tell his experiences to other people; but if he does so, he may lose all these merits and experiences and will find it difficult to win them back again. Furthermore, if one violates the Samaya Discipline, [Tantric Precepts], he will also lose the experiences and gains earned during his devotions. If this happens, he should think that all experiences, including the meritorious ones, are illusory —without self-entity, like rainbows — and should not cling to them, but contemplate on the truth of Sunyata. He should repent the fault of not keeping his inner experiences secret, and should determine not to tell anyone about them except his Guru in the future. If he has violated some of the Samaya rules, he should confess and recite the Mantra of Vajrasattva as restitution, and also apply to his Guru for new initiations, or pray to the Patron Buddha to initiate him once more. He should truly renounce all wordly glory, pride, and clingings, and determine to develop his meditation as a true yogi should.

If one follows the basic teachings of the Dharma, and practices in accordance with these instructions, he should not meet too many hindrances. However, for those of lower capacities and those who practice too vigorously, many hindrances of prana, nadi, and bindu, will arise. To overcome them one may refer to my other volume, *The Red Book of Heat Yoga.* [See the translator's note, p. 62.]

Those who take Dumo Yoga as their regular and constant practice should keep certain special rules. In order to preserve the warmth, the yogi should, during any meditation period, practice the breathing exercises at least a few times, and always visualize the Dumo-fire. He should be afraid of [neither heat nor] cold; even in bitterly cold weather he should never wear furs or very thick clothing, and should never go nude even in hot weather. He should not blow out a candle or fire, nor drink or eat extremely cold food.

In order to preserve the blissfulness, the yogi should make great efforts to retain his Tig Le; he should never lose it under any circumstances. Nor should he eat ginger, chili, pepper, garlic, spoiled fish or meat, or any kind of extremely sour, salty, or rich food. He should not stay too close to a fire or expose himself to the hot sun; nor should he sit on the ground without a cushion under him, walk barefoot, sleep during the day, or indulge in any activity that will cause much sweating.

To sustain his deep contemplation, he should live in solitude and renounce all meaningless activities.

THE EXPERIENCES AND MERITS OF DUMO YOGA PRACTICE

Because capacities and Karma vary greatly from person to person, it is difficult to generalize about the various experiences and merits produced by Dumo Yoga. One individual may have attained a great deal of "merit," but still may not have had many experiences; with another person, this may be reversed. It is also difficult to predict the definite sequence of the various experiences that a yogi must go through. Nevertheless, we shall now discuss briefly some of the more important effects of Dumo Yoga. In the foregoing pages we have discussed the signs, or experiences, of the taming of prana and the burning of Dumo-fire; now we shall discuss another significant topic, namely *the experiences that one has when the Prana-Mind is concentrated in the different Cakras.*

[According to the Doctrine of Tantra,] the nadis of each of the Five Cakras take the various forms of the special key-syllable [bija] of each Cakra. The five key-syllables, or to be more accurate, the five different forms taken by the nadis, are symbols or "expressions" of the five main desire-passions of man, namely lust, hatred, ignorance, pride, and envy. So in the course of Dumo practice, when the yogi concentrates on these Cakras, his Prana-Mind also gathers there. The concentration of Prana-Mind on these key-syllables will spontaneously stir up the desire-passions which the bijas represent. As a result, the yogi will feel all the great passions, such as *lust, hatred, doubt, pride, etc., arising freely and without his own volition.* All kinds of distracting and distressing thoughts and sicknesses will arise, thus impeding his devotion. Because of the concentration of Prana-Mind in the Cakras, he will also have a variety of delusory visions in dreams, in meditation, or in the waking state. This is when he should pray, repent, cultivate the Bodhi-Mind, strengthen his spirit of renunciation, and observe Sunyata in order to conquer these hindrances. He should also practice bodily exercises to untie the nadi-knots in the different Cakras. He should know that all these hindrances are actually helps, and good signs of his devotion, indicating that he is difinitely making progress in the Path. Thus, he should congratulate himself and gladly accept the challenge.

Having tamed the pranas and nadis, if the yogi can hold and gather the pranas of the Five Elements from their normal locations and lead them into the Central Channel, the Five Signs of Night — smoke, mirage, glow of the firefly, lamplight, and the light of the Unborn Void — will emerge; then, as he continues to hold the Five Pranas, the Signs of Day — moonlight, sunlight, "thunder-light," rainbow-light, and the light of sun and moon together — will emerge in turn. In some cases, many spots or motes of light will appear. These make, altogether, the so-called "Ten Signs."

If the pure essence of the pranas, nadis [?], and bindus can be gathered in the Five Cakras, the white, red, blue, yellow, and green Buddha Lands will appear. Also, if the Prana-Mind can be gathered in the mysterious nadis [?], the twenty-four secret holy places,[31] and the Yidams, Dakinis, and Guards[32] will also appear . . . .

He who can fully master the Five Pranas, or hold them in their respective Centers, will gain the following merits:

His body will become sturdy, his skin smooth, his face radiant and robust, and he will be full of energy at all times; even a high, thick wall cannot impede him.

He who can gather and hold the red and white Tig Les in the Central Channel, will gain the following three benefits:

(1) He can radiate beams of light from his body, and

also stand in the [sun]-light without casting a
shadow;

(2) Make his body vanish;

(3) Work various kinds of miracles.

He who can bring the Prana-Mind and the pure Essence
of the Five Elements into the Central Channel can:

(1) Transform stones into gold;

(2) Walk upon water without sinking;

(3) Enter fire without being burned;

(4) Melt a snow mountain with his Dumo-heat;

(5) Travel to a far-distant cosmos in a few seconds;

(6) Fly in the sky and walk through rocks and mountains . . . .

The scope and depth of the merits shown above vary
greatly according to the degree of proficiency in mastering
the Prana-Mind. The duration of the miraculous powers
[?] also varies greatly; if the yogi cannot hold the Prana-
Mind, these merits will also vanish.

Because the nadis and Tig Les are purified, the yogi
can work all kinds of miracles; because the Tig Le is stabilized and lifted [to the upper Cakras], the yogi can halt
a flowing river; because the Prana-Mind is concentrated,
he can hypnotize men by staring at them; because the Fire
Element is controlled, he can stop the sun in its course . . . ;
with the power of the nadis, he can produce wealth and
innumerable jewels; with the power of prana, he can attract
men; and with the power of Tig Le, he can attract Non-men
[Devas, ghosts, and demons] . . . .

Although one can procure all these benefits and merits, he should know that they are all illusory as rainbows, having no self-entity. He should never be conceited because of these powers, but try to overcome the Eight Worldly Gains[33] and concentrate upon the self-illuminating Mahamudra without distraction, for this is the only way to further one's Realization . . . .

In brief, the practice of Dumo Yoga enables one to realize the unborn Mahamudra Wisdom, to attain freedom from all clingings and ignorance, to untie all the Samsaric nadi-knots, to transform all Samsaric nadis into Wisdom-Nadis, to purify all karmic pranas and transform them into the obstruction-free Wisdom-Pranas, to purify all defiled Tig Les and transform them into the Tig Le of Bliss, and to attain the Two-in-One Rainbow Body of Perfect Buddhahood.

2. INSTRUCTIONS ON THE ILLUSORY-BODY YOGA

First, the yogi should complete all the preliminary practices, such as meditation on the transiency of life, on the sufferings of Samsara, on renunciation, on Compassion, on Bodhi-Mind, and so forth; then, in each period of meditation, he should devote a third of the time to Dumo practice. He should remind himself that it is to benefit all sentient beings that the Sambhogakaya [the glorious and divine Body] of Buddhahood is sought and the Illusory-Body Yoga now practiced. He should then pray for blessing and help to the red Sambhogakaya Guru with his consort [Yum],[34] sitting in the Throat Center . . .; he should think that all objects in the outer world — the houses, towns, mountains, rivers, men, animals, and all the organs and senses of the body — are merely manifestations of a confused mind and have no true existance or self-entity: they are like mirages, magic, dreams, bubbles, shadows, and dew, . . . for in reality they do not exist. He should think that all things that arise dependently [*pratitya-samutpada*] are like echoes and reflections, without the slightest self-substance, and then should continue to ponder on echoes and reflections; to think that all dharmas are momentary and fleeting like dew and bubbles; to visualize how the dews disappear with the rising of the sun and how bubbles vanish as the water flows by . . . . He should think that not even for a split second can things remain unchanged — that all dharmas are like rainbows, beautiful but unreal, and will soon vanish into nought . . . . In this manner he should meditate on Maya and Voidness. Even after this meditation he should continue observing the truth and play of Maya until he can eradicate all deep-rooted clingings.

[The foregoing practice is the foundation or preparation of the Illusory Body Yoga.] Now we shall discuss the practice itself, in two sections:

(1) The Impure Illusory Body Practice

(2) The Pure Illusory Body Practice

(1) INSTRUCTION ON THE IMPURE ILLUSORY-BODY PRACTICE

Standing before a mirror, observe the reflection of your own body — looking at the image for some time — and consider how this image is produced by a combination of various factors — the mirror, the body, light, space, etc. — under certain conditions. It is an object of dependent-arising [*pratitya-samutpada*] without any self-substance — appearing, yet void. Then observe the appearance of the image, together with its clothes and ornaments, and consider whether you are pleased or displeased with it; again feign to burst into anger, fight against yourself, and observe whether you are affected by it. Practicing thus, you will discover that all pleasures and displeasures are illusory and subjective, created by one's own mind, and so your clingings will be greatly reduced.

To practice the meditation on echoes, you should go to a place where they can be produced. Then shout loudly many pleasing and displeasing words to praise or malign yourself, and observe the reactions of pleasure and displeasure. Practicing thus, you will soon realize that all words, pleasant or unpleasant, are as illusory as the echoes themselves. If you can practice this meditation successfully, you will soon become indifferent toward both praise and blame, and you will attain Liberation . . . .

Until you can equate pleasure and displeasure, joy and pain, gain and loss . . . you should continue to meditate on illusoriness in a quiet place or in solitude. After this you can go to a village or town to practice among people and activities. If you find that you still react favorably or unfavorably to agreeable and disagreeable things, you should return to solitude and practice once more . . . .

(2) INSTRUCTION ON THE PURE ILLUSORY-BODY PRACTICE

In many of the instruction books of the Six Yogas, the meditation on the Self-Patron Buddha [Yidam] is not well explained. Although it is understood that one must first practice and achieve the Arising Yoga before he can practice the Perfecting Yoga, nowadays Tibetans seldom make this effort. [This is indeed very regrettable] because to visualize the Illusory Self-Patron Buddha is both a foundation for the Perfecting Yoga and a means to attain the perfect Sambhogakaya in the Bardo state. The visualization of the Self-Patron Buddha image of the Arising Yoga practice is therefore given below:

Procure a very clear painting of the Patron Buddha, place it [at an angle] between two mirrors, and observe the illusoriness of the three images. Use the picture as a support to visualize the Patron Buddha, until He appears as clear in your mind's eye as the sweetheart in that of a lover. The practicer is advised to visualize the complete image of the whole body all at once, and to hold it clearly as long as possible. After a while the vision will fade, and he should then visualize a given *part* of the body until it becomes extremely clear. He should start with the head and face; then the neck, the trunk, the limbs, and so forth, until the whole body becomes very vivid and clear.

As a person who has watched dancing for a long time can easily picture himself as the dancer, he who so observes a painting can also visualize it distinctly and with ease. A clear and stable vision can only be established through continual, regular practice. Interruption is fatal to the accomplishment of visualization.

Those who practice this exercise extremely well can see their vision even *more* clearly than the painting itself; those who practice moderately well can see it as clearly as the painting; and those not so well, more obscurely than the painting . . . .

Those who practice too hard will induce a great many distracting thoughts; if too loosely, will become drowsy. One should therefore adjust himself to different conditions and follow the middle way.

When the vision of the Self-Patron Buddha becomes very stable and clear, the yogi should go one step further, and identify the vision with Voidness. Visualization without a view of Sunyata [Voidness] is, at best, merely good imagination. Even the meditation on the illusoriness of the Patron Buddha Body — without a direct realization of Voidness — can, at best, produce a relative, but not the ultimate, Accomplishment. On the other hand, he who knows Voidness can at once realize the vision of the Patron Buddha as a projected mental illusion without the slightest self-substance. He sees that the appearance is the Void *per se,* and that there is *no need to identify it* with the Void . . .

During meditation the yogi should absorb the Patron Buddha vision into the self-illuminating Void without distraction. After meditation, he should try to keep the Awareness, and identify it with everything he meets . . . .

In brief, the vision of the Patron Buddha as projected in the Arising Yoga Practice is an expression of the Manifesting-Void Truth, and a symbol of illusoriness devoid of any substance or entity. If we use similes we may liken it to a magic apparition; to the moon's reflection in water; to a shadow without flesh and bones; a momentarily changing mirage; a dream projected by the mind; an echo born of dependent-arising; a phantasm without entity; a cloud continually changing shape; a rainbow, beautiful and vivid, but without substance; lightning, quickly appearing and vanishing; a bubble, suddenly arising and bursting; a reflection in a mirror, manifesting vividly but devoid of self-substance.

When the yogi can stabilize the Patron Buddha vision with ease and comfort, he should then expand the Yidam

Body to the size of the cosmos; shrink it to the size of a tiny mustard seed; and double it in a progressive series from one to millions. Then he should withdraw all these transformations into the original Body and meditate on that for some time. In daily activities he should identify all his experiences with the Buddha's Realm; houses and towns with the Mandala; the world with Buddha's Pure Land; all men with Buddhas and Bodhisattvas. He should think that all sounds are the chanting of Mantras; all thoughts a play of the Dharmakaya; all desirable objects and enjoyments, offerings to the Buddhas. In this way he should purify all the manifestations of Samsara and merge them with the Self-Illuminating Void.

* * *

To unfold the Four Voids or Four Blisses, the yogi should first bring the pranas into the Central Channel, and then from the Fourth, or Innate-Born Void, the Prana-Mind-made Illusory Body will arise. To achieve this, a blue *Hum* [ॐ] — the symbol of Prana-Mind — emanating five-colored rays, should be visualized in the Heart Center while the Vase-Breath is held. This is the way in which the pranas will be brought into the Central Channel and the signs of smoke, mirage, etc., . . . and the Lights of Revelation, Augmentation, and Attainment will emerge in turn. Meanwhile the *Hum* also dissolves into the Great Light. The yogi should then absorb himself in the Samadhi of Light as long as possible. Finally when he comes out of this Samadhi, he should project the Illusory Patron-Buddha Body with the Prana-Mind.

He who finds it difficult to do all these things properly should first concentrate on the blue *Hum* while holding the Vase-breath, and practice the Dissolving Process of that breathing.

A GENERAL REVIEW OF THE ILLUSORY-BODY PRACTICE

All things [dharmas] in both Samsara and Nirvana are devoid of self-nature and thus illusory. But the clinging, confusions, and discriminating thoughts of sentient beings make things appear to be real. To clear away this clinging and confusion, one should observe the void nature of all dharmas and learn the truth about maya.[35] This is the general principle of illusoriness.

The underlying principle of the Illusory-Body Yoga practice in the Tantras can be summarized in these words: Within the crude and karmic human body lies the pure essence of Buddha's Body concealed by men's clingings and confusions. Through the practice of the Illusory-Body Yoga Samadhi, these clingings and confusions will gradually be cleared away, and the illuminating-void Wisdom realized. As a result, the Samsaric pranas, nadis, and bindus are purified and the human body is transformed into the rainbow-like Illusory Body of Buddhahood.

The core of the Illusory-Body Yoga practice consists in unfolding the Innate Light and its successive projection of the Illusory Body through the Prana-Mind . . . .

During this practice, the yogi will feel strongly that nothing really exists. This experience will continue to deepen until one reaches full Enlightenment.

3. INSTRUCTIONS ON THE DREAM YOGA

The recognition of dream is the core of Dream-Yoga practice; to achieve this one must first remove all causes that becloud one's clear Awareness. The predominant causes that prevent Awareness, and their antidotes, are given briefly below:

(1) He who violates the Tantric Precepts will not be able to recognize dreams. In that case, the yogi should repent his transgressions and practice the Vajrasattva Mantra[36] to be cleansed from sins and to restore the Samaya Precepts. He should also try to obtain a new initiation either from his Guru or through prayer.[37]

(2) He who has little faith in his Guru and in the Tantric teachings will find it difficult to recognize dreams; in that case, he should try to strengthen his faith.

(3) He who is greedy for material gains will not be able to recognize dreams; in that case, he should give away his material belongings and stop clinging to this life.

(4) He who loses the Tig Le, or pollutes the body,[38] cannot recognize his dreams; so one should try hard to preserve the Tig Le and avoid associating with unclean persons, food, and places. If he must associate with them, he should perform the cleansing rituals for remedy.

(5) One cannot recognize dreams if his mind is full of distracting thoughts, or his yearning to do so is weak. In that case, he should live alone and try to strengthen his confidence and aspiration toward the Accomplishment.

(6) To think continuously in the daytime that all one sees, hears, touches . . . is in a dream, will greatly increase one's chances of recognizing dreams at night.

Before starting to work at Dream Yoga one should first complete the general preliminary practices, then spend one third of each period in practicing Dumo, and two thirds in visualizing the bija-syllables in the Throat Center — a good technique for generating dreams. First pray to the Guru sitting in the Throat Cakra for help in recognizing dreams at night; then visualize a four-petaled lotus in the Throat Cakra, in its center a white *Om* [᠊ᢌ᠋], on its front petal a blue *A* [᠊ᢖ], on its right petal a yellow *Nu* [ᢒ], on its rear petal a red *Ta* [ᢒ], and on its left petal a green *Ra* [ᢣ], — all very clear and vivid.

One may simplify this by only visualizing a red *Om* in the Center of the Throat Cakra and holding the Vase-Breath as long as he can; or he may mentally intone a long *Om* with each breath.

Some say that this should only be done during sleep. This is incorrect, because if it is treated in the daytime as the main meditation, quickly and easily the Prana-Mind will concentrate in the Throat Cakra, so that many more and clearer dreams will emerge. In addition, this practice will also help the prana to enter the Central Channel, and to unfold the Four Voids.

The yogi should think continuously in the waking state that all he sees, hears, touches, thinks, and acts upon, are in a dream. He should also avoid rich food or overeating, and not exhaust himself by strenuous activities. In short, he should try to combine the powers of prana, of strong will, and of other methods to recognize dreams.

The principal way to recognize dreams is to bring the pranas into the Central Channel for the unfoldment of the Four Voids. When this takes place, the yogi should identify them one by one, and then wait for the emergence of the dreams and try to recognize them. Elaboration of this practice will be given later.

The best time to observe dreams is between dawn and sunrise, because this is when food has been digested and rest completed, drowsiness is not heavy, and the mind is comparatively clear. But those who only sleep lightly can also practice this during the night.

The yogi should use a thin quilt, a high pillow, and lie on his side. Before falling to sleep, he should strengthen his confidence and determination to recognize dreams at least seven or as many as twenty-one times. He may visualize the four Key-syllables in the Throat Center for a while, and then concentrate solely on the red *Om* while gently holding the Vase-Breath.

A long and continuous sleep should be avoided; instead, one should try to sleep for many short periods. Each time one wakes up he should review whether he has successfully recognized his dreams during the preceding sleep. If not, a sincere prayer should be made before he sleeps again.

If after all this one still cannot recognize dreams. he should sit up and observe the objects in the room — the chair, table, bed, clothes, pictures . . . , and think that they are all visions in a dream. With this feeling he falls asleep once more.

He who cannot recognize dreams because of extreme drowsiness, should visualize a sparkling red *Om* in the Throat Center, radiating beams of light to fill his whole body and room, or a brilliant white Tig Le at the midpoint between the eyebrows. He who inclines to sleep very lightly should visualize a blue *Hum* or a blue Tig Le in the Secret Center . . . .

He who has diligently practiced all the above instructions, but still cannot recognize dreams, should retire in solitude, strip off all his clothing, jump, dance, and run in the nude, and shout loudly, "This is a dream! A dream!" He should also go to the edge of a dangerous cliff, look down into the abyss, and do the same. If he still cannot recognize dreams, he should be ashamed of himself and pray hard to his Guru and Patron Buddha. Then he should visualize in the Throat Center a [circle of] sharp blades rotating faster and faster, going up and down the entire body like a buzz-saw — slicing it into pieces and ashes — and offer them to the Buddhas and to hungry sentient beings. Then he should meditate on Mahamudra without discriminating thoughts . . . .

He who can only recognize dreams occasionally and momentarily, but not constantly, will find his practice rather inefficient. This is especially true in the case of sudden awakening immediately after the recognition of dreams. If so, the yogi should repeatedly warn himself against this tendency and strengthen his desire to remain in the dream state. Even if awake, he should not open his eyes, but try to keep on dreaming, or concentrate on the Heart or the Secret Center.

The yogi should investigate carefully what causes rapid awakening from dreams — if too much tension, he should relax more; if noise, he should sleep in a quieter place; if cold or heat, he should wear more or fewer clothes; and so forth. Some instructions say that to visualize oneself sitting between a red and white Tig Le — the positive and negative forces — will help. It is also said that to visualize a blue *Hum* in the Throat Center, while holding the Vase-Breath, will also help . . . . In brief, the yogi should always try to find out why he cannot recognize dreams, and then take the appropriate remedial measures. For example, if too drowsy, visualize a red or white Tig Le in the Throat, or in the midpoint between the two eyebrows, radiating brilliant light; if too alert, or too easily awakened, visualize a blue or black Tig Le in the Heart or the Privy Center; if the dreams are not clear, visualize a red Tig Le in the Throat Center, radiating a bright light covering all the nadis in the entire body . . . .

When the yogi has a frightening dream, he should guard against unwarranted fear by saying, "This is a dream. How can fire burn me or water drown me in a dream? How can this animal, or devil, etc., harm me?" Keeping this awareness, he should trample on the fire, walk through the water, or transform himself into a great fireball and fly into the heart of the threatening devil or beast and burn it up . . . .

The yogi who can recognize dreams fairly well and steadily, should proceed to practice the *Transformation of Dreams*. This is to say that in the Dream state, he should try to transform his body into a bird, a tiger, a lion, a Brahman, a king, a house, a rock, a forest . . . or anything he likes. When this practice is stabilized, he should then transform himself into the Patron Buddha Body in various forms, sitting or standing, large or small, and so forth. Also, he should transform the things that he sees in dreams into different objects — for instance, an animal into a man, water into fire, earth into space, one into many, or many into one . . . . He should exercise the various supernatural powers, such as shooting fire from the upper body or water from the lower body, trampling on the sun and the moon, or multiplying his body into millions and billions to fill the entire cosmos . . . .

One of the main purposes of Dream Yoga practice is to assist one to realize the Illusory Body in the Bardo state, and in this lifetime. To achieve this, one must first recognize the Four Voids of Sleep;[39] then from the Fourth or the Innate Void, he instantaneously projects the Prana-Mind-made Illusory Body of the Patron Buddha in a Mandala, and then dissolves the Mandala and the Patron Buddha into the great Void once more. This is, briefly, the Arising and Dissolving process practiced in the Dream Yoga.

After this the yogi should practice the *Journey to Buddha's Lands* as instructed below:

Visualize oneself as becoming the Patron Buddha, and instantaneously, like a shooting star, arrive in the Heaven of Indra, or some other Samsaric Heaven; observe the place before returning. When this is stabilized, one should then journey to one of the Buddha's Pure Lands, such as the Pure Land of Vairocana, of Amitabha, or the like. This, too, is done in a split second. Reaching Buddha's Pure Land, he should make obeisance and offerings to the Buddha and listen to His preaching . . . .

In the beginning, the visions and experiences are not very clear, but one should firmly believe that what he sees in the dream is the real Pure Land itself, for both Samsara and Nirvana are, after all, but dreams; practicing thus, the visions will become clearer and clearer . . . .

If one asks, "Is there any difference between the Illusory Body Yoga and Dream Yoga practice?" the answer is that they are basically alike, but the Dream Yoga should be regarded as supplementary to the Illusory Body Yoga. One is used to generate the Illusory Body, and the other to further or perfect it. One should also know that the

Illusory Body which arises from the Light in the Waking state is much deeper and more subtle than that of dreams. But both Yogas should be practiced to supplement each other; for in this way, the clinging-of-time manifested in the dichotomy of Dream and Waking states can eventually be conquered. The combined practice of these two Yogas can lead one to purify the habitual-thoughts of Samsara, to realize that all things are manifestations of the mind, and that mind is devoid of self-entity, like dreams; to know that both Samsara and Nirvana are unreal mirages, and that they bind nothing and liberate nothing; to cleanse oneself of all the crude and subtle, pure and impure attachments; and finally to unfold the magic-like Sambhogakaya of Buddhahood.

4. INSTRUCTIONS ON THE LIGHT YOGA
How to Recognize the Light

The steps taken in the preliminary practice to remove all impediments and gather all favorable conditions for recognizing the Light, are the same as in Dream Yoga. But in addition, the yogi should eat good and nourishing food, massage his body, live in a very quiet place, preserve his Tig Le, and be gentle and relaxed at all times. In each period of meditation, he should spend one third of the time practicing Dumo, and two thirds practicing Light Yoga. He should first visualize a blue Vajradhara with consort sitting in his Heart Center, and pray to Him for the unfolding of the Innate Light; then he should visualize a blue *Hum* in the Heart Center and hold the Vase-Breath, or mentally intone a long *Hum* . . . then all the outer world dissolves into his body, the body into the *Hum,* the *Hum* into the Nada,[40] and the Nada into the great Void. He should meditate on the Void and hold his breath. Arising from this Samadhi, the yogi should again visualize the Illusory Body of the Patron Buddha, and so on . . . .

Some people claim falsely that this should only be done at night; but the fact is that if one practices this throughout the day, he will greatly increase the chance of mastering the Prana-Mind and will stabilize the revelation of the Light, so that it will be much easier for him to recognize the Light during sleep. Besides, great advantages will be added by holding the breath at the same time. To recognize the Light by other methods is very difficult; and the light so recognized cannot last very long . . . . He who follows this practice is certain to bring the pranas into the Central Channel and unfold the Four Voids . . . . This is, therefore, the most important practice of Light Yoga.

HOLDING THE LIGHT DURING SLEEP

Those who can unfold the Four Voids in turn by gathering the pranas in the Central Channel during the day can also do so during sleep if they concentrate on the *Hum* in the Heart Center immediately before falling asleep.

The best time to "hold" the Light is not [in the middle of the] night when sleep is very heavy, but at dawn, or whenever the sleep is light; and the best posture is to lie on the side, with both knees bent.

Here, the two essentials of Light Yoga practice are to visualize the five key-syllables on the five lotus petals in the Heart Center, and to hold the breath.

Before falling asleep, the yogi should think [over and over], twenty-one times, that he *must* recognize the Innate Light when it emerges after the stages of Revelation, Augmentation, and Attainment. Then he visualizes his whole body dissolving into the *Hum* and the *Hum* into the Light, and concentrates upon it. When he feels slightly sleepy, he concentrates on the *A* [ཨ]; when quite sleepy, on *Nu* [ཟ]; when very sleepy, on *Ta* [ཏ], when almost falling asleep, on *Ra* [ར], and as he falls asleep [or becomes unconscious], on *Hum* [ཧཱུྃ].

In the beginning the yogi may find it difficult to visualize the last two syllables, because he tends to fall asleep immediately after concentrating on the first three; but through repeated practice he can gradually do so. He who cannot remain aware in the unconscious state of sleep, should practice hard in the daytime in order to gain more Samadhi power. This will enable him to remain aware in the unconscious state and see some of the Light . . . .

Some instructions say that if one still cannot recognize the Light, he should abandon sleep for three days and nights and then try again . . . .

He who can unfold in turn the Four Lights or Voids, i.e., the Lights of Revelation, Augmentation, Attainment, and the Innate-Born, can eliminate both crude and subtle Samsaric thoughts and transcend the discriminating mind. Then he will see face to face the genuine Light-of-Sleep, as transparent and clear as a cloudless sky. This is the superb experience, or the perfect Light. Next to this is what we may call the "fair" experience, or the "lesser" Light, in which, although the yogi cannot recognize the Four Voids in turn or eliminate all Samsaric manifestations, he can overcome heavy drowsiness and discern clearly the transparent Illuminating-Voidness. Next to this is the "inferior" experience, in which the yogi can neither recognize the "perfect" nor the "lesser" Light, but experiences a clear and transparent mind in the state of sleep before dreams arise . . . . This is called the experience of the "corresponding Light."

If through daytime practice one has attained a stable Samadhi, its power will carry through day and night, including the states of sleep and dream. In that case, the yogi will not [as a rule] dream; and if he does, he can recognize it at once. But some Gurus say that this is not the Light-of-Sleep, but only an experience of Samadhi in the state of sleep. This may be true, but if one can so practice, he really can increase his chance of recognizing the Light and will soon see the "lesser" Light.

Although there are many methods of holding the Light, the foregoing instructions are quite sufficient for the purpose; the yogi should follow the particular one most helpful to him . . . .

COMMENTS ON THE FOUR VOIDS

The Four Voids, Four Lights, or Four Blisses, are the core of the Light-Yoga experience. They are induced by gathering of the pranas in the Central Channel in the daytime practice of the waking state. He who can do so, should concentrate particularly on the Fourth Void, or the Innate Light. The method for recognizing these Four Voids is as follows:

During the Light-Yoga practice at night, the yogi should first concentrate on the *A* on one of the lotus petals in the Heart Center. Through this practice the pranas of the Five Elements will gather in the Central Channel and the signs of smoke, mirage, firefly-light, etc., will emerge in turn. When he feels sleepy, he should concentrate on the *Nu*, whereupon more pranas will be gathered, crude discriminating thoughts will dissolve, and the Initial Void, or Light-of-Revelation, will emerge; he will then experience a feeling as though seeing bright moonlight in a cloudless sky. When the yogi becomes sleepier, he should concentrate on the *Ta*, more pranas will be gathered, all subtle discriminating thoughts will dissolve, and the Second, or the Extreme Void — otherwise called the Light-of-Augmentation — will emerge; now he will experience a feeling as though seeing sunlight in a cloudless sky. When he feels very sleepy, he should concentrate on the *Ra*, whereupon all the pranas will be gathered, the majority of the most subtle discriminating thoughts will dissolve, and the Third, or Great Void — otherwise called the Light-of-Attainment — will emerge; he will then experience a feeling as though seeing all-embracing darkness in a deep and cloudless firmament. Finally, as the yogi falls asleep [or becomes unconscious] while concentrating on the *Hum*, all the pranas of the Attainment and all the most subtle discriminating thoughts will dissolve, and the Fourth, or Total Void—otherwise called the Innate Light — will emerge; then he will experience a feeling as though seeing the vault of the clear sky at dawn, and all the Three Defilements of sun, moon, and twilight will leave him . . . . These are the Four Voids, or Lights-of-Sleep which the yogi must recognize and practice.

At the start, one may not be able to recognize all these Four Voids, but with continual and persistent practice, he will eventually do so. Those who are not proficient in "holding" the Four Voids, should practice the Yoga during light sleep; those who are, should practice it in deep sleep. He who is not yet well versed in holding the Light through the regular process will find it difficult to do so in reverse, i.e., from the Innate Light to hold the Third, the Second, and then the Initial Light. The regular process is therefore basic and very important.

If one is forced to emerge from the Samadhi of Light by the agitation of prana, he should concentrate on the *Hum* in the Heart Center to restabilize the Samadhi. If this does not help, he should then try to meditate on the "lesser" Light. If he is forced to emerge from the "lesser" Light, he should then try to practice the Illusory-Body-of-Dream. But to do this properly, he must be able to gather the pranas in the Central Channel and to unfold the Four Voids in the daytime practice. Only when one reaches this stage can he completely hold the Light at night. Less advanced yogis may recognize the First or Second Light, but to do so with the Third, and the Innate Light, will be extremely difficult for them.

If before going to bed one arouses a very strong desire to hold the Light, and concentrates on the *Hum* in the Heart Center radiating brilliant light—filling the entire body—he will stand a good chance of seeing the "lesser" Light. In a state of light sleep without dreams, he will see the Mind-nature as illuminating and yet empty—transparent without obstruction. His awareness is as clear as though he were awake. Nevertheless, he cannot eliminate distracting thoughts, and sometimes his illuminating Awareness also coemerges with dreams. If this occurs, he should still concentrate on the *Hum* and try to keep the illuminating Awareness in order to stabilize the Light. He who cannot recognize the Light during deep sleep should not become discouraged, but instead should try again to become aware, and gradually he will succeed. If because of the agitation of prana, some dreams arise, he should identify these visions with the Patron Buddha and His Mandala, then try once more to dissolve them into the great Void . . . .

One should know that the "lesser" Light is not the real Light-of-Sleep; the latter is the Fourth, or Innate Light devoid of all distraction and discriminating thoughts, whereas the former is only a superficial Light mingled with discriminating thoughts and distractions. But if one can stabilize and strengthen this "lesser" Light, he will eventually succeed in holding the Innate Light. At present, many yogis in Tibet can only reach the state of holding the "corresponding" Light; even those who can practice well can only hold the "lesser" Light. It is therefore extremely important to know this difference . . . .

COMMENTS ON THE THREE FUNDAMENTAL LIGHTS

Light, according to the teaching of Tantra, can be classified into three groups:

(1) The Light-of-Origin
(2) The Light-of-the-Path
(3) The Light-of-Fruition

The Light-of-Origin, or of Reality, is the Innate Light that exists at all times regardless of whether one is aware of it or not. The Light-of-Sleep and the Light-of-Death belong to this class. The Light-of-the-Path is the direct realization of Sunyata, or the Four Lights or Voids which unfold when the pranas enter the Central Channel. It can also be called Non-discriminating Wisdom—a realization of the Unborn Void that transcends the dualism of subject and object . . . . The Light-of-Fruition is the realization of the Two-in-One Ultimate Light, the perfect and complete Enlightenment of Buddhahood.

The Light-of-Sleep can also be divided into various groups: That which is recognized in deep sleep without "object-facing" is called the Light-of-Deep-Sleep; that which is recognized with crude and subtle objects is called the "lesser" Light-of-Sleep, and so on.

As instructed before in the Dream Yoga, one should observe whether he is confident and able to master the Bardo. He should ask himself, "With my present Realization can I master the Light-of-Death when the time comes?" If he can master the Four Voids of Sleep, he can be assured of recognizing the Four Voids at the time of death. For him, death is a very helpful step on the Path.

So, by the practice of this Light Yoga, Samsaric clingings and disriminations will be purified and the Self-Illuminating Wisdom realized. With the Wisdom Fire of the Innate Light, one can destroy all impure habitual thoughts, merge the Son- and Mother-Light into one, and embrace all in the great totality of the Inborn Light . . . . One will then attain the perfect Dharmakaya and Rupakaya,[41] and until the end of Samsara he can, without the slightest effort, help all sentient beings in a countless number of ways.

5. INSTRUCTIONS ON THE BARDO YOGA

THE PHENOMENON OF DEATH

To practice the Bardo Yoga one should first understand the basic principles of Bardo, information on which can be found in other sources. Wide reading on this subject from various Sutras and Tantras is needed.

I will now briefly describe the phenomenon of death:

(1) When the Skandha of Form[42] begins to dissolve, one feels weak to the point of exhaustion. When the Earth ele-

ment begins to dissolve, the body becomes desiccated; when the organ of sight dissolves, one cannot move the eyeballs or see clearly; when the element of the Great-Mirror-Wisdom[43] begins to dissolve, one's mind becomes very dim and dull . . . .

(2) When the Skandha of Feeling begins to dissolve, one feels sluggish and numbed; when the element of Water dissolves, the secretions within the body stop; when the organ of hearing dissolves, one cannot hear; when the element of the Wisdom-of-Equality dissipates, one cannot distinguish between joy and pain.

(3) When the Skandha of Perception begins to dissolve, one cannot see any outer objects; when Fire-element dissolves, one cannot digest; when the nose begins to fail, the upper prana slows down and becomes irregular; when the sense of smell dissolves, one cannot distinguish odors; when the element of the Wisdom-of-Observation dissipates, the dying cannot recognize relatives standing round them.

(4) When the Skandha of Action dissolves, one cannot do anything; when the element of prana dissipates, the Ten Pranas will return whence they came; when the organ of taste dissolves, the tongue shortens and thickens; when the sense of taste fails, one cannot distinguish different flavors; when the element of the Wisdom-of-Activity dissolves, one can neither act nor will.

According to another Scripture, the following information concerning death is given:

(1) When the Earth element dissolves into Water, the outer sign is that one cannot move his body, feeling as if he were losing all support and about to collapse. He wants

to cry out, "Please help me to stand up!" The inner sign is that the consciousness appears like whirling clouds of smoke.

(2) When the Water [element] dissolves into Fire, the outer sign is the drying up of all secretions; the inner sign is that the consciousness manifests as shifting mirages and all the thirty-three discriminating thoughts of anger[44] subside.

(3) When the Fire [element] dissolves into the prana, the outer sign is a drastic reduction of bodily heat, while the fingers and toes become numb and cold; the inner sign is that the consciousness manifests as a dim spark of firefly-light, and the forty discriminating thoughts of lust subside.

(4) When the prana dissolves into the consciousness, the outer sign is that the dying person's exhalations become very long and his inhalations very short. The inner sign is that the consciousness appears as clear and steady lamplight, and all the seven discriminating thoughts of ignorance subside.

. . . . According to the Scriptures, these signs of death may appear one after the other or all at once, depending on the individual.

When the subtle elements dissolve, the dying person will have the following experiences:

(1) When the consciousness dissolves into the Light-of-Revelation, he will see light like that of the moon in a cloudless sky.

(2) When the Light-of-Revelation dissolves into the Light-of-Augmentation, he will see a streak of light—reddish-blue in color like the dawn.

(3) When the Light-of-Augmentation dissolves into the Light-of-Attainment, he will experience complete darkness and lose consciousness.

(4) This unconscious state will again dissolve into Light, and a transparently clear Void like a cloudless sky at dawn—transcending all subtle defilements of the previous three stages—will emerge. This is the true Light-of-Death, or the Innate Light . . . .

When the different elements have dissolved, one after another, the element of prana will finally dissolve into the consciousness at the Heart Center. Then the white Tig Le in the Head Center will descend, the red Tig Le in the Navel Center will rise, and the two will join in the Heart. When the red and white Tig Les have completely merged, the Light-of-Death will appear. Every sentient being in the Six Lokas [Realms] will see the Light-of-Death once at the end of each life, but unfortunately, he will not be able to recognize and hold it . . . .

THE EMERGENCE OF BARDO

. . . . Then, in the reverse process, from the Light-of-Death the Attainment, Augmentation, and Revelation will arise in turn. When the dormant prana begins to move, the Light-of-Attainment will emerge; and immediately thereafter, the Lights of Augmentation, and of Revelation will follow. Then the eighty discriminating thoughts will arise, and as a result, all the delusory manifestations of Bardo will appear . . . .

A controversial question often arises here: "What do the Bardo-dweller's body and face look like?" According to the Asangha brothers, they take the shape of the next incarnation. But others say they are similar to those of the previous incarnation. According to the Gurus of the Succession, however, in the early stages of Bardo the Bardo-dweller's face and body resemble those of the previous incarnation; then they gradually fade away until, in the latter stages of Bardo, they assume the appearance of the coming incarnation. This theory is not only reasonable, but accords with the Scriptures. Many Sutras clearly indicate the existence in the Bardo state of the "Body-of-Habit," shaped after the previous incarnation. The great *Commentary* on the *Tantra of Kalacakra* also agrees. This point will become quite clear if we take dreams as an example. In them, because of habitual thinking, we do not change face and form. By the same token, one's habitual thoughts will continue to sustain his form in the early Bardo, and only in the later stages, when the habitual thoughts of the previous life have faded away, will a new bodily form, shaped like that of the coming incarnation, appear.

A Bardo-dweller has all organs complete and can travel anywhere without obstruction except to the place where he is destined to incarnate again. He has some Samsaric superpowers, feeds on the fragrance of food, and can see other kindred Bardo-dwellers.

If the Bardo-dweller is destined to be born in the miserable realms, he will have a vision of profound darkness, or of a black, rainy night . . . . If he is to be born in a happy realm, he sees a white light brilliant as the moon . . . .

Another scripture says: "Those who are to be born in Hell will see all things colored blackish-brown, like burned wood; those to be born in the realm of Hungry-Ghosts will see smoky colors; those destined for Heaven will see golden light; those to be born in the Heaven-of-Form (*rapadhatu*) will see white . . . and those to be born in the Formless Heaven (*arupadhatu*) will have no experience of Bardo— they will incarnate in the Formless Heaven immediately after death . . . . It is said, however, that those sentient beings in the Formless Heaven destined to be born in the lower realms, will again experience Bardo . . . .

When the Earth element is disturbed, the Bardo-dweller hears the thunder of explosions; when the Water element is disturbed, he hears the boom of ocean waves; when the Fire element, he hears the roar of a burning forest; and when the Wind element, he hears the high scream of a hurricane . . . .

The Three Poisonous Passions—lust, hatred, and ignorance—cause the Bardo-dweller to have various kinds of fearful visions in white, red, and black—his confused. habitual thoughts projected as fearful ghosts and devils approaching to harm him.

A Bardo-dweller is said to possess these qualities:

(1) His body offers no resistance and casts no shadow; and in a split second he can travel to many lands.

(2) Sentient beings in other realms cannot witness his acts.

(3) He is clairvoyant and telepathic.

(4) He sees neither sun, moon, nor stars.

(5) He watches the Innate Spirit[45] record in detail all the good and sinful deeds committed in his previous life.

(6) Although he sees food, he cannot enjoy it unless it is offered or dedicated to him.

Although the above descriptions have been given, it is difficult to accept them as definite or invariable, because the Karma of individuals is never the same, and the manifestations also vary greatly. In many ways the Bardo-state is like the Dream-state—very unstable and uncertain.

The maximum length of the Bardo-life is seven days, but if within this time the Bardo-dweller has not reincarnated, he "dies" or falls into a swoon to be reborn immediately in the second Bardo. This process can be repeated seven times—totaling forty-nine days.

The Bardo-dweller falls in love with the place where he is to be reborn as soon as he sees it.

He who is to be born through wetness or warmth will be attracted by fumes and odors.

He who is to be born in worm or egg form will conceive great lust and hatred toward both of his parents when he sees their intercourse. He who is to be born as a man will love the mother and hate the father, and [as a woman,] vice versa. As soon as this lust and hatred arise, the Bardo-dweller will immediately fall into a swoon, and without realizing it, will be reincarnated . . . .

He who is to be born in one of the heavens will see the splendid, heavenly mansions, with male and female angels, and desire them . . . .

He who is to be born in the miserable realms will see many fearful visions and try desperately to avoid them.

If he escapes to a cave, a pit, or a tree he will be born as
an animal; if he escapes to an iron house he will be born
in Hell . . . .

When the Bardo-dweller dies he will also go through the
four stages of the dissolving process, i.e., the subsidence
of pranas into the Revelation, the Augmentation, the Attainment, and the Innate Light. Then the reversing process
will begin—from Innate Light, to Attainment, to Augmentation, to Revelation, to the eighty discriminating thoughts,
to the elements of prana, of fire . . . until the body-mind
complex has been completed.

THE OPPORTUNITY OF BARDO

At the time of death, when the Son- and Mother-Light
merge, all the subtle defilements of discriminating thought
will subside. At this time an advanced yogi who has
mastered both the Arising and Perfecting Yogas can attain perfect Buddhahood and its merits at once. One who
is fairly advanced, but can practice the superb Mahamudra
day and night, can also hold the Light of Death; and then,
when the visions of Bardo appear, can utilize them to
further his Realization . . . .

Some people claim that it is possible, even with slight
merits and preparations, to realize the Dharmakaya at the
time of death, and the Sambhogakaya and Nirmanakaya in
the Bardo state. This statement is baseless and contrary
to the Scriptures: Those who make it do not realize that
to hold the Light, even for a short while, is extremely
difficult; and that to remain unconfused by the bewildering
and fearful visions of Bardo while utilizing them as a means
to further one's devotion, is even harder. This is clearly

demonstrated by the fact that even we, the living, have great difficulty in recognizing the Light-of-Sleep-and-Dreams here and now. Even if we can recognize the Light and the dreams, we cannot hold them firm, nor can we master and transform dreams as we please . . . But this criticism does not imply a denial that those who prepare and practice during their lifetimes will benefit by it at death and in Bardo.

All manifestations of this world are, in fact, those of Bardo, and all Samsaric existences are those of Bardo. The period between birth and death can be called the "Bardo-of-Life-and-Death"; from the time of falling asleep till awakening the "Bardo-of-Dream"; from death till reincarnation, the "Bardo" *per se.* In these three Bardos, the Dumo and Illusory-Body Yogas, the Light and Dream Yogas, and the Bardo and Transformation Yogas, respectively, should be stressed for practice.

In both the sleep and waking states, one should think that all he sees, hears, touches, and acts upon is in the state of Bardo. He should know that continued and repeated practice of this instruction is an excellent preparation for Bardo.

Many Gurus have said, "In practicing the Bardo Yoga, one should not forget the instructions for a second, even if he is pursued by seven ferocious Tibetan dogs. When the time of death draws near, he should offer his property and belongings to the Three Precious Ones,[46] give charity unsparingly, cut off all attachments, observe strictly the Samaya Precepts, and repent all transgressions and sinful deeds . . . . Also he should seek reinitiation from his Guru or from Buddha to reinstate the Samaya Precepts if he ever broke them. He should pray sincerely to his Guru and

Patron Buddha for help in holding the Light-of-Death and the Illusory Body in Bardo, and rely on his spiritual friends to remind him of the instructions at his death-bed."

The most advanced yogi should, at the time of death, practice the Dissolving Yoga, and concentrate on the Self-illuminating Essence to merge it with the Light-of-Death; then from the Light he should try to raise the Prana-Mind-made Perfect Sambhogakaya and Nirmanakaya.

Those very advanced yogis who have reached the Fourth Stage of Mahamudra can surely merge the Mother- and Son-Light at the time of Death. Then all the ties of the Karmic body, of manifestations, and of mind, will be cut; and all the merits of Buddhahood will be completed. Their minds will become the Dharmakaya, their bodies the Body-of-Wisdom, and their Land the Land-of-Perfection-and-Purity.

Fairly advanced yogis should also practice in the same way as the most advanced. If they can succeed in this, they will bypass the Bardo stage and reach a more advanced Bhumi [stage] in the Path. If not, they should pray earnestly to be born in Buddha's Pure Land, and apply the teaching of the Transformation Yoga . . . .

Those inferior yogis, who can neither hold the Light-of-Death nor the Illusory Body, should try to alert their mindfulness, and with definite understanding and unshakable confidence apply the Instructions to meet the challenge of death and Bardo. He who cannot utilize the opportunity of death and Bardo to gain Liberation will be forced by Karma to incarnate once more in Samsara. To prevent this, the following instructions should be applied:

When the Bardo-dweller comes to a place most attractive to him, he should visualize it as the Mandala of his Patron

Buddha. When lust and hatred arise because of seeing the intercourse between man and woman, he should alert himself and think that this is the Third Initation of the Father and Mother Buddhas. He should accept the Bliss-Void experience, and observe that both lust and hatred are illusory and void.

Thus stressing the view of Sunyata, he may free himself from Samsara forever. If the Bardo-dweller can do this successfully and escape reincarnation in the first seven days, he will find no difficulty in doing the same during the next seven days and after. He will be born in the Pure Land of the Patron Buddha and complete his devotions in the Path.

If the Bardo-dweller wants to be born in Buddha's Pure Land, he should develop a strong desire to incarnate there. This is of vital importance. Then he should apply the instruction of the Transformation Yoga, and in a split second he will be born in the Pure Land . . . .

The benefit of Bardo Yoga can be summarized thus:

(1) The Dharmakaya can be realized at the time of death,

(2) the Sambhogakaya in Bardo, and

(3) the Nirmanakaya at the time of incarnation.

This is also called the Path that leads to the accomplishment of the Buddha's Trikaya.

6. INSTRUCTIONS ON THE TRANSFORMATION YOGA

Transformation Yoga is a teaching devised to deliver one's consciousness to the Buddha's Pure Land, or to a higher realm of birth. For those advanced yogis who can hold the Light-of-Death and the Illusory-Body-of-Bardo, this

Yoga is not necessary. But for those who have not yet
reached the advanced stages, it is extremely important. He
who has mastered the Arising Yoga, and to some degree
the pranas and nadis, and the Mahamudra view, is best
qualified to practice this Yoga. Those who cannot, should
at least have great faith in this teaching, believe strongly
in the law of Karma, and thoroughly understand the meaning and process of this practice. They should also be
reasonably proficient in holding the Vase-Breath in the
Dumo Yoga as mentioned before.

How to Practice the Transformation Yoga

The visualization and exercise of the Transformation
Yoga should be practiced as follows:

In the Self-Yidam Body [Self-Patron Buddha Body],
visualize the Central Channel and eight *Hum* syllables, each
covering one of the eight exits of the body to prevent the
escape of consciousnes from these Gates[47] .... Then visualize the Patron Buddha sitting in the sky before and
above you, and a blue *Hum* in your Heart Center radiating
five-colored light. Next, hold the Vase-Breath and apply its
power to shoot the *Hum* up through the Central Channel
to the Gate of Purity [a tiny opening in the Center on
top of the head,] and at the same time shout "Hig!"
loudly to strengthen the force of the "shot." Now keep the
Hum at the Gate of Purity for a second and then gently
mutter "Gha!" to bring it down and back to the Heart
Center. Repeat this seven times before stopping; then
resume the practice. After a few rounds, shout "Hig!" seven
times running, and shoot the *Hum* out of the body to enter
the Patron Buddha's Heart in the sky above. Then repeat—

gently and in a lower tone—"Gha!" seven consecutive times, thus returning the *Hum* to your own Heart Center.

He who does this four times a day will, in a few days, have the following experience: The top of the head will itch badly and feel hot, and in its center a lump will rise and secrete a form of yellowish liquid . . . . If these symptoms occur, he should know that they are the signs of accomplishment. After this he should stop, only repeating the practice once or twice a month; but he should frequently make a strong vow to be born in Buddha's Pure Land, and strengthen his confidence and desire to go there.

Application of the Transformation Yoga

When all signs of death appear and nothing more can be done to prolong life, the Transformation Yoga should be applied. He who does so before he is due to die commits a great sin and will be damned . . . .

The technique of this Yoga at the time of death is the same as that given before, except that the upper part of the Central Channel and the Gate of Purity should be visualized as immensely large and unobstructed. Now visualize *Hum* in the Heart Center and, pulling up all your strength, shout "Hig!". At once the *Hum* shoots out from the Central Channel, passing through the Gate of Purity, and in a split second reaches the Heart of the Patron Buddha in the sky before you. *If at this moment you feel everything becoming very dark, the prana gushing out, and the top of the head itching or painful, know that this is a sure sign that you are about to leave the body for Buddha's Pure Land.* If no such signs appear, bring the *Hum* down, rest, and try once more. When these signs appear, continue shouting "Hig!" twenty-one to twenty-five times, and you will definitely be born in the Pure Land.

The friends, relatives, or whoever attends the dying person, should also assist him at this critical time by reminding him of the instructions of the Transformation Yoga, strengthening his confidence and faith, and praying for him . . . .

Those who have not had an opportunity to practice this Yoga during their lifetimes can try as follows:

When death approaches, pray, make offerings, repent, and state wishes before the Buddhas. Arouse the Bodhi-Mind, renounce all evil thoughts, and cut off all attachment. Lie on your right side—facing the West—bend both knees, and place the left leg over the right one. The right hand should rest under the right cheek and the left hand on the left leg. Then, arousing an earnest desire to be born in the Buddha's Pure Land, apply the Transformation Yoga instructions. He who does not know them should be briefed by someone who does. If the latter is not available, simply concentrate on the Heart of the Patron Buddha standing before and above you in the sky, and continuously shout "Hig!" twenty-one times, thus flinging your consciousness into the Buddha's heart . . . .

If one gently rubs the dying person's head and repeats "sMan.Lha"—one of Buddha's names—the Eight Bodhisattvas will come to lead the dying one's consciousness to Buddha Amidha's Western Paradise . . . .

He who sees a dying animal should repeat "Ratnakuta"—another name of Buddha—and the consciousness of the animal will be born in a higher realm . . . .

Those who cannot realize the Light-of-Death and the Illusory-Body-of-Bardo, but rely on the Transformation

Yoga to be born in a higher realm, can be divided into three groups: Well-endowed yogis who incarnate in Buddha's Pure Land can easily attain Ultimate Enlightenment there; average ones can incarnate in a place where the Dharma and the Vajrayana prevail, and so in few lifetimes will also reach Buddhahood; inferior ones, by means of this Yoga, can avoid the great pains of death, escape from the fear of Bardo, and incarnate in a happy place; so eventually they, also, will earn Liberation . . . .

Epilogue

He who practices this profound teaching of the Six Yogas should never be contented or self-satisfied because of minor good experiences gained in meditation. Instead, he should practice with diligence and modesty to the end of his life . . . . If one lacks determination and perseverance, he should meditate on the transiency of life and the sufferings of Samsara . . . . If he is selfish and egocentric, he should meditate on Compassion, good will, and the Bodhi-Mind . . . .

When practicing the Six Yogas one should never abandon the basic Dharma meditation, such as reciting the prayer of "Taking in Refuge," meditating on Compassion and the Bodhi-Mind, repentence, prostrations, dedications, and so forth . . . . He should practice these for at least one or two periods a day. As to the main meditations of the six Yogas he should practice them four to six times a day—when awake, working at Dumo and the Illusory-Body Yogas when asleep, at the Light and Dream Yogas.

He who has not mastered the Dumo Yoga can neither cause the prana to enter, remain, and dissolve in the Central Channel, nor unfold the Four Voids or Four Blisses, nor project the Illusory Body from the Light. As a result, he cannot practice the Dream and Bardo Yogas properly . . . . This is why Dumo is considered to be the most important practice of the Six Yogas.

One should, therefore, spend at least half or one third of his time in practicing Dumo, even when his main work is on the other Yogas. Once in a while he should also practice the Bardo and Transformation Yogas to refresh his memory of them . . . .

THE CONJUNCTIONS OF THE SIX YOGAS

[Since Tantrism is based upon the view of the identity of Samsara and Nirvana, the sublimation of the Passion-Desires, and the unfoldment of the Innate Trikaya], the practice of the Six Yogas can thus be "conjoined" or "associated" with the three Passion-Desires and Buddha's Trikaya in a number of ways. The practice of the Dumo and Illusory-Body Yoga in the waking state can be "associated" with the element of lust; that of the Light and Dream Yogas with ignorance; that of Bardo and the Illusory Body [?] with hatred.

To absorb oneself in the Innate Light is to associate with the Dharmakaya; to project from the Light the Illusory Body made by the Prana-Mind is to associate with the Sambhogakaya; to dissolve the crude elements of the body in the Central Channel and transform them into a Mandala is to associate with the Nirmanakaya . . . .

At the time of death, to absorb oneself in the Innate Light is to associate with the Dharmakaya; to project the

Illusory Body in the Bardo state is to associate with the Sambhogakaya; and to incarnate in various places and forms is to associate with the Nirmanakaya . . . .

Again:

Sleep corresponds with the Dharmakaya, dream corresponds with the Sambhogakaya, and waking corresponds with the Nirmanakaya . . . .

There are many other ways to "conjoin" or "associate" the Six Yogas with the Trikaya and Passion-Desires, but the above are sufficient to illustrate the general principle.

. . . . Those who have mastered both the Arising and Perfecting Yogas and aspire to attain Perfect Buddhahood in this life should practice the "Secret Act." However, nowadays in Tibet, there are few yogis who can do this. It is therefore unnecessary to elaborate this topic here. Those who are interested in knowing about it should consult other sources. According to the Gurus of the Whispered Succession, he who practices these "Secret Acts" not only should accomplish the Arising and Perfecting Yogas, but also practice the act itself in accordance with the Hinayana and Mahayana Precepts. He should utter no worldly remark, but frequent cemeteries, forests, remote mountains, and all other deserted places to practice the Tantric offerings and acts. Like a wounded animal, his mind has no interest in this world; like a lion, he goes anywhere without fear. He acts like the wind in the sky and attaches no value to this life. His mind is objectless like the Void; his actions are free like those of a lunatic, without discrimination . . . .

THE ACCOMPLISHMENTS OF THE SIX YOGAS

There are two kinds of accomplishments that one can expect to achieve through practicing the Six Yogas, the one mundane and the other transcendental. The former includes (A) the Four Performances, and (B) the Eight Siddhis [accomplishments].

THE MUNDANE ACCOMPLISHMENT

The Four Performances are:
(1) The attainment of power to prevent calamities and misfortunes for oneself and others.
(2) The attainment of power to increase merits and good fortune.
(3) Power to attract desirable things.
(4) Power to overcome all hindrances and evils.

The Eight Siddhis are:
(1) The attainment of a mysterious sword that can grant all one's wishes.
(2) The attainment of magical pills with miraculous powers of healing.
(3) The attainment of a wondrous eye-salve which bestows clairvoyance.
(4) The power of rapid walking.
(5) A magic elixir which transforms age into youth.
(6) Power to take part in the act with goddesses.
(7) Power to conceal one's body among crowds.
(8) Power to pass through walls, rocks, and mountains . . . .

These worldly accomplishments can be attained by the practice of the Arising Yoga alone, but the Transcendental, or Supreme Accomplishment only through the combining practice of both the Arising and the Perfecting Yogas . . . .

THE TRANSCENDENTAL ACCOMPLISHMENT

We shall now discuss briefly the various stages of Transcental Accomplishment.

The four stages in the Path are:

(1) He who has entered the Path and stabilized the practices and experiences of both Yogas is considered to have reached the first stage—the Stage of Gathering Provisions.

(2) He who can lead the Prana-Mind into the Central Channel and bring forth the "Down-coming Four Blisses" through the descent of the pure element of Prana-Mind, experiences the Bliss-Void directly, increases immensely the mundane merits of prana and nadis, and is said to have reached the second stage—the Stage of Anticipation.

(3) He who can pull the pure element of Tig Le up through the Central Channel, bring forth the "upgoing Four Blisses," stabilize the Tig Le in the Head Center, untie in turn the knots that bind the Central Channel, . . . clear all blockades in the Six Cakras, and eliminate one after the other the twenty-one thousand, six hundred karmic pranas, is said to have reached the third or fourth stages—which include the Stages of Initial Enlightenment and of Further Enlightenment, i.e., from the First Bhumi [stage] to the Twelfth.

(4) He who can purify the most subtle pranas, nadis, and bindus, transform the physical body into the Rainbow-Body, purify the thirty-two nadis and the eighty discriminating thoughts—thus unfold-

ing the wondrous thirty-two signs and eighty splendid forms of the Buddha's Body—is said to have reached the Perfect Buddhahood of the Thirteenth Bhumi of Vajradhara. Because His Prana-Mind is one of Wisdom, and because the *A* and *Ham*[48] syllables are perfectly united, He attains the Ultimate Two-in-One Sambhogakaya of Buddhahood. That which in Him expresses the Non-differentiation of Compassion and Voidness is called the Dharmakaya; that which in Him expresses the infinite Bliss and Glory is called the Sambhogakaya; that which in Him expresses the infinite forms and plays produced for the benefit of sentient beings is called the Nirmanakaya. The identity, or unity of these Bodies is called the Body of Dharmadhatu [Totality]. With these Four Bodies He will set in motion the Wheel of Dharma to deliver all sentient beings till the end of Samsara . . . .

NOTES

1 Trikāya: The Three Bodies of Buddha, i.e., the Dharmakāya — the Body of Reality; the Sambhogakāya — The Body of Enjoyment; and the Nirmāṇakāya — the Body of Transformation. The Dharmakāya is the embodiment of Śūnyatā, that which is primordially unborn. It is transcendental and beyond all attributions and designations. The Sambhogakāya is the divine manifestation of the Dharmakāya — the-Body-of-Splendor-and-Glory revealed only in the realm of Buddha's Pure Land. The Nirmāṇakāya is the Transformation Body incarnated in various worlds for the benefit of sentient beings.

2 Vajradhara (T.T.: rDo.rJe.hChań.): According to the tradition of Tibetan Tantrism, Buddha Vajradhara is considered to be the first Buddha to have given forth all of the Tantric teachings.

3 The Three Yogas: These probably refer to the Yogas designed to tame the body, mouth, and mind.

4 The Supreme Accomplishment: perfect Enlightenment, or Buddhahood.

5 Gambopa: the chief disciple of Milarepa, a great scholar and yogi who, in the 12th century, propagated the Ghajyuba School in Tibet.

6 Dumo (T.T.: gTum.Mo.; Skt.: Caṇḍālī): the "mystic" fire or heat produced in the Navel Center during the Heat Yoga practice.

7 Bardo (T.T.: Bar.Do.): the intermediate state between death and rebirth. According to Buddhism, this is a very important state which provides not only a good opportunity for Liberation and Enlightenment, but also is like a crossroad to the Bardo-dweller whose fate and fortune depend much upon it. See the section on Bardo Yoga.

8 Pith-Instructions (T.T.: Man.Ñag. [or] gDams.Ñag.): This may also be rendered as "Key-Instructions," which consist of the essence of the Tantric teaching conveyed from Guru to disciple, usually in a very simple, precise, yet practical form.

9 Six Yogas: the Yogas of Dumo-Heat, of Illusory Body, of Dream, of Light, of Bardo, and of Transformation.

10 Lord of Secrets: another name for Vajradhara; some say it is another name for Vajrapāni.

11 Dākinīs (T.T.: mKhah.hGro.Ma.; lit.: female sky travelers): the Tantric Goddesses who protect and serve the Tantric Doctrine. They are not invariably enlightened beings; there are many so-called Worldly Dākinīs (T.T.: hJig.rTen.mKhah.hGro.Ma.) who are still bound in Samsāra.

12 The Two Yogas: In the *Anuttara Tantra,* the "Supreme Tantra," there are two major practices: one is the Arising Yoga (T.T.: sKyed.Rim.) and the other is the Perfecting Yoga (T.T.: rDsogs.Rim.). The former, which can also be translated as the Yoga of Growth or of Creation, is a preparation for the latter, and stresses the concentration and visualization practices. Its main features contain the following steps:

(1) Visualizing all objects and the self-body as dissolving into the great Void.

(2) Visualizing in the Void a bīja seed transforming itself into an image of the Self-Patron Buddha.

(3) Visualizing the Self-Patron Buddha Body in its entirety, including the Three Main Channels and the Four Cakras.

(4) Visualizing the Mandala and identifying all manifestations with Buddhahood.

(5) Reciting the Mantra of the Patron Buddha and applying a specific visualization for a special yogic purpose.

(6) Visualizing all objects, including the Self-Patron Buddha Body, as dissolving into the bīja in the Heart Cakra, and the bīja again dissolving into the great Void.

(7) From the Void again projecting the Self-Patron Buddha and the Mandala.

This Yoga stresses visualizations and the basic yogic and spiritual training, in order to lay the groundwork for the Perfecting Yoga practice. But since this is all done with conscious effort through the "mundane mind," it cannot be considered as transcendental in nature, and is designed merely as a preliminary practice for higher Yogas.

The Perfecting Yoga is the advanced Tantric Yoga practice, its main aim being to lead the karmic prāṇas into the Central Channel and transform them into the Wisdom-Light, thus realizing the Dharmakāya. Then from the Dharmakāya, the yogi is taught to raise the Sambhogakāya and Nirmāṇakāyas. In the Perfecting Yoga group, the Heat and Illusory-Body Yogas are the two primary ones — the Light, Dream, Bardo, and Transformation Yogas being subsidiary.

13 The Six Elements: earth, water, fire, air, space, and consciousness.

14 Ālaya Consciousness (T.T.: Kun.gShi.Nam.Çes.), or the Store Consciousness — that which preserves or "stores" all memories and habits. It is also called the Fundamental Consciouness, Primordial Consciouness, the Consciousness of Ripening Karma, and so forth. Both Yogācāra and Tantric Buddhism stress the importance and study of this Consciouness. When one reaches Buddhahood, it is transformed into the so-called "Wisdom of the Great Mirror."

15 Seven Consciousnesses: the Consciousnesses of Eye, Ear, Nose, Tongue, Body, Discrimination (mind), and Ego-clinging. These, with the Ālaya, make a total of eight.

16 Because of the present unavailability of Tibetian reference books, the translator has no way of identifying the names of these "eighty types of distracting thoughts."

17 Revelation, Augmentation, and Attainment (T.T.: sNañ.Ba., rGyas.Ba., [and] Thob.Ba.): These are the three stages in which the Three Voids successively emerge and the eighty discriminations and Desire-Passions successively subside during the process of the "Dissolving of Prāṇa-Mind." This can take place before sleep, at the time of death, and upon the prāṇa's entering the Central Channel. See the section on Light Yoga.

18 Foundation, Path, and Accomplishment (T.T.: gShi.Lam.hBras.-Bu.): These three terms are frequently used in Tibetan Tantric

texts. Foundation (T.T.: gShi.) implies the basic principles of Tantric Buddhism; the Path (T.T.: Lam.) is the practice, or way of action which is in conformity with the principle of the "Foundation"; Accomplishment or "Fruit" (T.T.: hBras.Bu.) is the full realization of the principle óf the "Foundation." For example, the Foundation of the Six Yogas is based on the conviction that the innate Buddha-nature, without which no practice can possibly bring forth the Trikāya of Buddhahood, lies within one's own body-mind complex. Foundation is, therefore, the cause, the seed, or the potentiality of the Trikāya within all sentient beings; the Path of the Six Yogas is the practice set up within the framework of this basic principle; and the Accomplishment is the full realization of the Trikāya.

19 Demchog: (T.T.: bDe.mChog.; Skt.: Śaṃvara): an important Tantric deity of the Mother Tantra.

20 Arising Yoga (T.T.: sKyed.Rim.): See Note 12.

21 Gate of Purity (T.T.: Tshaṅs.Bu.; Skt.; Brāhmarandhra): the hidden "aperture" on the top of the head. This is the only Gate or exit by which man's consciousness can leave the body and be born in Buddha's Pure Land.

22 The Three Channels: the Central (T.T.: dBu.Ma.), the Right (T.T.: Ro.Ma.), and the Left Channel (T.T.: rKyaṅ.Ma.). These are the three mystic Channels, or nāḍīs, in the body. All three are situated in the central part of the body, running parallel to one another. The Right Channel is said to correspond to the solar system, the Left to the lunar system, and the Central to the unity of the sun and moon. The Right and Left Channels are regarded as Saṃsāric ones, and the Central as the Channel that leads to Nirvāṇa. A clear visualization of these three Channels is a prerequisite for the practice of the Six Yogas.

23 The Four Cakras (T.T.: rTsa.hKhor.bShi.), or the Four Centers, are situated in the head, throat, chest, and navel, respectively, and cojoin with the Central Channel. The Head Cakra is also called the Center of Great Bliss; the Throat Cakra, the Center of Enjoyment; the Heart Cakra, the Center of Dharma; and the Navel Cakra, the Center of Transformation.

24 Tig Le (T.T.: Thig.Le.; Skt.: Bindu), meaning "dot" or "drop," when used in Tantric texts signifies the "essence" of the vital energy, namely, male semen and female "blood." In a broader sense, Tig Le seems to denote all secretions within the body, especially those of the endocrine system. Tig Le is also an equivalent of Bodhi-Mind when the latter is used in the Tantric sense.

25 Prāṇa-Mind (T.T.: Rluñ.Sems.): See the Foreword and its Note 2.

26 By using a finger to block the left nostril and inhaling through the right, then reversing this process and inhaling through the left, one will soon discover that in one of the nostrils the breath flows more freely than in the other. According to "Tantric physiology," there are only six periods within each twenty-four hours in which both nostrils carry the breath evenly. This is said to be due to alternations of the "prāṇa-changes" in the Navel Cakra. Judging by the time and force of the breathings through both nostrils, the yogi can foretell many important events affecting himself and the world. This art is fully elaborated in Garmapa Rangjhang Dorje's book, *The Profound Inner Meaning* (T.T.: Zab.Mo.Nañ.Don.) [unavailable in translation at this time. Tr], and other sources.

27 Bīja syllables (T.T.: Sa.Bon., meaning "seed") are the essence, or the main symbols of a deity, of a Cakra, of an element, or the like. It is believed that by working on a bīja one can awaken or master the element it represents.

28 Ever-stable Vase-Breathing: a soft and gentle type of Vase-Breathing; its main feature is to put a constant but gentle pressure on the lower part of the abdomen.

29 The essence of Mahāmudrā practice is clearly given in Part I, especially in Lama Kong Ka's THE ESSENTIALS OF MA-HĀMUDRĀ PRACTICE, which is, in fact, the core or pith of the verbal instruction of Mahāmudrā. Drashi Nanjhal's *Comprehensive Survey of Mahāmudrā Meditation* is a very scholarly work, also a voluminous one, and, so far, has never been translated into any European language. The main purpose and theme of this work is to provide a theoretical background to Mahāmudrā in

the light of the Prajñāpāramitā. It is the translator's opinion, however, that no higher or profounder teachings on Mahāmudrā practice can be found than Lama Kong Ka's instructions, together with the *Song of Mahāmudrā* and the *Vow of Mahāmudrā*. Vast indeed is the Tibetan literature, but the highest teaching itself is always simple and precise. (Garma C. C. Chang)

30 The Four Bliss-Wisdoms, or the Four Bliss-Void Wisdoms (T.T.: bDe.sToñ.Ye.Çes.): In general Mahāyāna Buddhism, the "Wisdom-of-the-Void" is often stressed; but the "Bliss-Void Wisdom" seems to be exclusively of Tantric provenance. In the Six Yogas, the "Four Voids" and the "Four Blisses" also seem to be interchangeable.

31 These are the so-called "twenty-four gathering places" of Ḍākinīs and Tantric yogis in India.

32 Yidam (T.T.: Yi.Dam.): the Patron Buddha, chosen by one's Guru during Initiation, to whom one prays, and upon whom one relies. In the Arising Yoga practice, the yogi visualizes his physical body as becoming that of the Patron Buddha — who is, in fact, a yogi's *reliance* in all his yogic practices. Dākinīs, (T.T.: mKhah.-hGrol.Ma.), meaning lady-sky-travelers, are Tantric goddesses who play extremely important roles in all Tantric acts. Guards (T.T.: Sruñ.Ma.) are the Tantric gods or spirits who protect the Doctrine, and guide and serve the yogis.

33 The Eight Worldly Gains, or Eight Worldly Winds: the eight "winds" or influences which fan the passions, i.e., gain, loss; defamation, eulogy; praise, ridicule; sorrow, joy.

34 Yum: the Mother Buddha.

35 Māyā: illusions or delusions. Māyā is the doctrine that the manifestations we·experience are all illusory or delusory, without true existence.

36 Vajrasattva Mantra: a famous and important Mantra consisting of one hundred syllables; its main function is to purify sins and to remove all spiritual hindrances. Almost all Tibetan Lamas recite this Mantra in their daily prayers.

37 If a qualified Guru is not available, the yogi can pray to the Buddha directly and receive the Initiation from Buddha through visualization and prayers.

38 If a Tantric yogi contacts forbidden persons and things, or goes to "defiled" places, he will expose himself to the danger of pollution, thus hindering his yogic progress.

39 The Four Voids of Sleep: the four successive unfoldments of the Void taking place immediately before or after sleep. They are: the Initial Void, the Extreme Void, the Supreme Void, and the Innate Void. The difference between these four Voids consists in the degree of their clarity and "thoroughness."

40 In the dissolving of the *Hūm* word, the last small spot perceivable — the final, tiny point left in the "dissolving process" of the *Hūm* after the vanishing of the Tig Le (Thig.Le.) — is known as the "Nāda." See the following drawing: [$\int$ Nāda]. It is also said that "Nāda" is the self-born mystic sound which is not produced through the collision of two objects.

41 Rūpakāya: the Body of Form, which refers to both the Divine Body (Sambhogakāya) and the Transformation Body (Nirmāṇakāya) of Buddhahood.

42 The Skandha of Form (lit.: the Aggregation of Form), actually refers to all matter, objects, or anything that is composed of the various elements. The "Five Skandhas," a very frequently used term in Buddhist literature, was originally given to refute the idea of absolute being, of an indivisible ego, a self-entity, and the like.

43 The Great-Mirror Wisdom: This term should not be taken literally here, because ordinary sentient beings cannot be said to have any of the Five Wisdoms of Buddhahood as given in this section. The reason for this expression is that, according to Yogācāra Buddhism, when one reaches Buddhahood his five Consciousnesses (those of Eye, of Ear, of Nose, of Tongue, and of Body) become the Wisdom-of-Performance, or Activity; his mind, or the Sixth Consciousness, becomes the Wisdom-of-

Observation; his Ego-Consciousness, the Seventh, the Wisdom-of-Equality; and his Ālaya Consciousness, the Eighth, the Wisdom-of-the-Great-Mirror.

44 Here again, lacking the Tibetan reference books, the translator has no way of identifying these names.

45 Innate Spirit or Innate Ghost: This is actually a projection of one's own conscience, transfigured in the form of a spirit, who records all one's good and evil deeds and presents them to the Lord of Death (Yama).

46 The Three Precious Ones: the Buddha, the Dharma, and the Saṅgha.

47 The Eight Gates: the two ears, two eyes, nose, mouth, anus, and privy organ.

48 *A* is the bīja of the Navel Center, symbolizing the positive element; *Ham* (pronounced Häm) is the bīja of the Head Center, symbolizing the negative element. These two are also called the red and white Tig Le, or Bodhi-Mind.